# SURGERY
# AND
# RECOVERY

*I wish you
health & peace*

*Kay*

As a Family Practice physician, I find *Surgery and Recovery* a much needed addition to the world of medicine. I firmly believe that most patients who need surgery "insulate" themselves with denial, fear, and a lack of knowledge of what the proposed surgery will do for and to them. Despite educational efforts by surgeons, a great deal of what they say falls on deaf ears because of the patient's fear. This book is a great resource for patients, something tangible to which they can refer over and over. My office will not be without a supply.
—Faith B. Fritsch, D.O., Family Medical Services

\* \* \* \* \*

Today's healthcare system relies heavily upon the patient and family for pre and post-operative care. Knowledge and understanding of the surgical process by the consumer is essential for a successful recovery. Ms. Olson's book encourages the patient and support person to advocate for their physical and emotional needs. It guides the consumer to wellness with information and strong self-care promotion.
—Mary Jane Cook, B.S.N., CCRN, Surgical Intensive
   Care Unit, Michigan Capital Medical Center

\* \* \* \* \*

With insight and sensitivity, Kaye Olson offers practical suggestions for dealing with the fears and other emotional concerns of surgical patients and their families. She anticipates their questions and addresses specific needs with sound advice. Recognizing the importance of a holistic approach to healing, Olson provides a helpful set of well-researched techniques for dealing with the psychological and physical aspects of healing and recovery.
—Richard Dombrowski, Ph.D., Licensed Psychologist,
   Psychological and Family Therapist

\* \* \* \* \*

*Surgery and Recovery* is an immensely practical guide—the very best book I've ever read on the subject. Ms. Olson helps one

become informed and educated about surgery, which paves the way to make a powerful difference in the success of the surgery and healing process. Highly recommended!
—Charlene A. Schaar, Consumer, Retired School Teacher

*  *  *  *  *

Many patients feel stripped of their dignity upon admission for surgery. *Surgery and Recovery* directs patients and families, then opens the door to communication on needed issues. Better-prepared patients are at less risk and experience a safer path to recovery and wholeness. Feeling good about the total surgical experience can be a positive chapter in one's life if the patient is well-informed, in control of choices, and treated with respect.
—Susan Cole, R.N., Nurse Educator,
  Memorial Healthcare Center

*  *  *  *  *

This book is an excellent tool for patients facing surgery. It provokes the patient to seek information from the healthcare system. By reading *Surgery and Recovery*, patients become empowered, educated, and active participants in their own health care which results in a smoother and more successful surgical experience.
—Diane Southwell, B.S., M.A., Health Education Manager,
  Blue Care Network Mid-Michigan & East Michigan

*  *  *  *  *

As a pre-surgical nurse, the most relaxed patients are the ones who have had all of their questions answered so they understand the procedure that is about to be performed. Olson's informative book is an excellent reading if surgery is in your or a family member's future. *Surgery and Recovery* offers questions to think about and prepares the patient, through necessary steps, for a smoother surgical experience.
—Sue Neuder, R.N., Sparrow Out-patient Care Unit

*  *  *  *  *

*Surgery and Recovery* helps to alleviate much of the stress and anxiety associated with a major medical treatment. However, the book's most important contribution may be for males who suffer needlessly because they are reluctant to ask questions or discuss medical procedures. An individual facing surgery needs to know what to expect in order to retain personal control and create a positive healing atmosphere. This book provides a sense of control and a means to overcome feelings of helplessness. The personal stories of courage and determination serve as positive guides for total healing.
—Tom Nelson, Consumer, Community College Counselor

\* \* \* \* \*

At Michigan State University, we select references which reflect current research, communicate facts and information in an understandable format, and are a combination of statistics and believable examples. Olson's book is a winner on all of these accounts. Her carefully documented book is certain to attract multitudes within the university community who might be anticipating surgery or need information to advocate for a family member.
—Judy McQueen, M.A., Educational Program Coordinator, Michigan State University

\* \* \* \* \*

Surgery can often feel like a frightening leap into the unknown. This holistic guide gently, but realistically, leads the reader step-by-step to a much better understanding of the whole process. As a practicing family physician, I have counseled my patients on numerous occasions regarding impending surgery. Ms. Olson answers in a concise, yet compassionate way, the many issues that arouse concern in potential candidates for an operation. *Surgery and Recovery* is an excellent book to be read by people anticipating a surgical experience.
—Barry Saltman, M.D., Family and Community Medicine

\* \* \* \* \*

# Surgery and Recovery

## HOW TO REDUCE ANXIETY AND PROMOTE HEALTHY HEALING

KAYE OLSON, R.N., M.A.

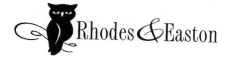

Rhodes & Easton

TRAVERSE CITY, MICHIGAN

This book is designed to give you general information on the surgical process, encouraging you to follow the advice of your surgeon and other experts addressed in the text and resources. The information is not intended to give specific legal, insurance, nutritional, or medical advice, nor should you substitute the information for medical advice or treatment.

 Published by Rhodes &Easton
121 E. Front Street, 4th Floor, Traverse City, Michigan 49684

Publisher's Cataloging-in-Publication Data
Olson, Kaye.
    Surgery and recovery: how to reduce anxiety and promote
    healthy healing / Kaye Olson—Traverse City, Michigan:
    Rhodes & Easton, 1998
        p.   cm.
    Includes bibliographical references and index.
    ISBN 1-890394-03-3
    1. Mental healing. 2. Surgery—Popular works. I. Title.
RZ400.047    1998
615.852  dc21      97-67641

00  99  98  ◆  5  4  3  2  1

Printed in the United States of America

*This book is dedicated to men and women facing surgery, recovering at home following an operation, or advocating for a parent or other family member.*

*May you feel enlightened, encouraged, and empowered by this guide, its resources, and the personal stories.*
*May the surgery and recovery process be safer and more successful.*

# CONTENTS

## PART III: Letting Go, But Taking Control

## PART IV: Homeward Bound

# FOREWORD

*A*s a surgeon, my philosophy is that knowledge and skills must be passed down to the next generation. That is why I have devoted my life to teaching—teaching patients—teaching medical students and residents.

To me, patient education has always been important. If patients understand their problems, why surgical operations are necessary to correct certain afflictions of the body, how these operations will be done, and what effects may impact their daily normal life activities, their fears may lessen and their chances for a smoother and more coordinated post-operative recovery will be increased.

To be able to educate patients about their medical problems, there should be a good patient/surgeon relationship based on open communication and trust. Patients must provide a thorough and accurate medical history to enable the surgeon to make the best clinical diagnosis; to order additional tests, if necessary; to confirm the diagnosis and plan the surgical operation; anticipate potential problems; and minimize post-operative complications.

Options regarding the management of a patient's surgical problem should be fully discussed, including the pros and cons, with the active participation of the patient and the family. Physicians should talk to patients in a manner that is supportive and in language that can be clearly understood.

The seeds of trust must be sown during the first encounter. If, for any reason, the patient exhibits a lack of trust, a second opinion should be requested.

Most patients want to be educated about their upcoming surgical operation and are groping for information to help themselves. All patients feel nervous; all patients feel stress.

There are many books published by prestigious medical institutions on the technical and various aspects of surgery, but I have not found a book that is solely focused on the needs of the patient. I believe that Kaye Olson's book fulfills that need.

Her guide offers practical information to patients, in a language that is easily understood, on a wide variety of essential topics, including insurance information. She helps patients to understand the surgical process, how to make the right decisions with surgical operations, and how to take responsibility during the recovery period.

With the right diagnosis and the right operation, the patient does well. With the wrong diagnosis and the wrong operation, the patient does poorly. Educating the patient and the family is one of the important keys to a successful outcome.

Rafael S. de los Santos, M.D.,
Professor of Surgery,
Department of Surgery,
College of Human Medicine,
Michigan State University,
East Lansing, Michigan

# INTRODUCTION

*M*ore than 50 million surgeries are performed annually in America. Men and women have a 50% probability of having an operation at some time in their lives. Your chance of being hospitalized this year is one in ten. Recently, an analysis of several hundred studies disclosed that when people psychologically prepare for surgery, the hospital stay is reduced by 1.5 days.

When surgery is suggested, people and families want information. This practical and comprehensive book eases the experience by walking the reader through the surgical process while emphasizing a safe and successful surgery. With this resource guide, the reader can also achieve a healthier recovery and take control of his or her life at a time when the world seems upside down. Adults advocating for an aging parent or family member, and professionals functioning in consumer advocacy roles, will also appreciate the information.

Designed as a "reader friendly" guide, this book organizes the information in four sections. The first part focuses on concerns confronting people when surgery is needed, from examining the insurance coverage to choosing the right surgeon. Other topics include: feeling the emotions, considering blood donations and advance directives, preparing the family, and organizing the home before the operation.

The second section presents ideas to prepare oneself mentally and physically for the operation and shows how to clarify information with the nurse, surgeon, and anesthesiologist. Surgical preparations and relaxation are also included.

In part three, the day of surgery and the hospital recovery period are discussed, from going through the admitting process to securing the going home instructions.

Within the final section, the recovery process at home is addressed, encouraging the reader to set boundaries, create a healing environment, build the blood back up (if needed), and to resume home, work, and social life slowly.

Six men and women describe their surgical experiences, weaving hope, strength, courage, and reality among the informational chapters, reinforcing the book's strategies for a successful operation. Throughout their personal stories, they present creative ways to manage the surgical process and reveal techniques and therapies that complement medical practices. Assertiveness, persistence in obtaining information, communication, a positive attitude, a strong belief system, visualization, and listening to the body are lessons demonstrated through the various experiences.

For enlightenment, the reader can use this guide in many ways: reading it in sequence, choosing the most important chapters, focusing on the "Keys for Taking Control" summary at the end of each chapter, doing the suggested activities, or concentrating on the stories.

A wealth of information in the back of this book awaits patients, family members, and advocates. The glossary of terms, self-help groups, national resources (including websites), bibliography, and index provide wonderful resources.

Surgery is a humbling experience—the essence of complete vulnerability. It transforms a man or a woman in full control into someone with little control. Regardless of the type of surgery, the experience impacts a person mentally, emotionally, physically, and spiritually. I know because I've been there too.

My surgeon said "We need to talk about a possible breast biopsy because I'm concerned with your left breast and the possibility of lobular carcinoma."

Cancer? Me? I froze. Nothing could have prepared me for what I was hearing.

He continued. "This cancer, which is increasing in women over 40, can't be diagnosed by standard breast screening, such as a mammogram, needle biopsy, or ultrasound."

He put my options out on the table and talked about each one thoroughly. Over time, the suspected problem could be watched through frequent breast evaluations in his office or the breast could be biopsied. He tossed the ball to me and said I should let him know what I wanted.

I don't remember driving home. Then reality hit. I got angry. He said I had a choice, but I really didn't have a choice. If I didn't have the biopsy, I might regret not finding a problem early on. If I did have the biopsy, I would know if I had cancer or not. Over the next 48 hours I struggled with the pros and cons. I chose the biopsy.

Since an abnormal mammogram eight years ago, my surgeon had been monitoring my breast tissue for any potential problem. I had complete trust in his judgement; we had a positive relationship. He had always explained my mammograms and exams extensively and had never failed to respond to my many questions. I also knew he was the best in the area.

The proposed surgery couldn't have come at a worse time. I was already scheduled for a major surgery in seven weeks. Before that, I needed to finish a hectic semester at the college, complete my scheduled speaking engagements, and take a trip to Greece that was already paid for. How could I fit a second surgery in? When? The "why me" and "why now" nagged at me, while anxieties kicked in.

I was drowning in overload due to other events in my personal life. I was still reeling from the deaths of two close family members; little did I know that my brother and father would also die in the next few months. My daughter was going through a divorce and I was trying to support her and the grandchildren. My life seemed unreal—this couldn't be happening to me.

My first priority was to get to the medical library where I reviewed the consumer information and medical sections. Over a six-hour period of time, I immersed myself in every medical article on lobular carcinoma, read the information, then copied each article to take with me.

As I hustled from the medical library, a calmness embraced me. Obtaining information had eased my fears. The medical articles matched what my surgeon was doing. As I consulted my nursing and physician colleagues, they, too, supported my decision. Slowly I became more comfortable with the decision to have surgery.

After both surgeries (which were negative for cancer), I bathed myself in self-nurturing activities. I created a healing environment at home and soothed myself with natural sounds to relax and hasten recovery.

Two weeks after my major surgery, I started a journal. I wrote about my surgeries, what had been helpful, how things could have been different, and what was important for holistic healing. That journal grew into this book.

As a nurse practitioner, I have always been a strong patient advocate. With a psychology background, I've always been intrigued with the mind's power over the body, especially in healing. My devotion to patient education, which served me well in my clinical nursing role, now extends into my other professional roles. As a stress consultant throughout the Midwest and instructor at Lansing Community College, Lansing, Michigan, my push for education continues.

There is never a good time for surgery. Emergency and elective surgeries present themselves like uninvited guests whenever they choose. But, if surgery is necessary, it is crucial to be informed so you can make the right decisions. There are many ways to take control of your life, or advocate for a family member, at this vulnerable time to ease this inevitable process. Knowledge is power.

*—Kaye Olson*

# ACKNOWLEDGMENTS

*A* book blossoms with the support of many people. Special gratitude goes to Linda R. Peckham, Professor of English, Lansing Community College, Lansing, Michigan, for her enthusiastic coaching and feedback over the years.

For writing the Foreword, deepest appreciation is expressed to Rafael S. de los Santos, M.D., Professor of Surgery, College of Human Medicine, Michigan State University, East Lansing, Michigan. His words demonstrate a passion for patient education and a belief that a "team approach" brings a more successful surgery.

Recognition goes to Edward J. Madara, Director of the American Self-Help Clearinghouse for providing self-help groups. Thanks to all of the national organizations listed in the resource section for helping surgical patients.

I am indebted to Judy, Pat Sorg, Ken Shapiro, Linda Peckham, Christina DeLand, and Barry Stearns for sharing their surgical experiences so others could learn from them. Their revealing lessons of hope, personal strength, and creative coping are invaluable and weave a thread of reality among my informational chapters.

My heartfelt appreciation to Bernie S. Siegel, M.D., author of *Love, Medicine and Miracles*, guru of hope, health, humor, and healing; and Don R. Powell, Ph.D., profound advocate of self-care, Founder and President of the American Institute for Preventive Medicine, for their support.

For those who reviewed the manuscript and offered endorsements, I express my sincere appreciation to Charlene A. Schaar; Tom Nelson; Faith B. Fritsch, D.O.; Mary Jane Cook, B.S.N., R.N., CCRN; Richard Dombrowski, Ph.D.; Susan Cole, R.N.; Barry Saltman, M.D.; Sue Neuder, R.N.; and Diane Southwell, B.S., M.A.

To Kay Babbitt, R.N. and Gladys Stauffer, L.P.N., surgical nurses, thanks for your gentle critique and ideas to make the book so timely. For other professionals, Suzanne Hollister Saltman, Mary Laing, Connie Sutton, N. Jean Green, Marilyn Boyd, and Ruth Fienup, thanks for your constructive ideas to improve the information.

With persistence and gusto, Judy McQueen reviewed the text and brought objectivity to the script. Thank you, Judy. For library support, gratitude is expressed to Suzanne L. Sawyer-Burleson, Electronic Information Services Librarian, and Anne Rau, Reference Librarian.

Thanks to Joan Tirak, Nina Machtel, Norma and Palmer Bollinger, Laura Fawcett, and Jane Idzkowski for on-going support and other friends, colleagues, and relatives who asked how I was doing throughout this journey.

To Erik, my husband, I'm grateful for your computer expertise on the days, evenings, and weekends of hard work. Special thanks to my daughters, Barbara Olson and Debra Meredith for their help. And to my brother, Karl Gruetzman, thank you for the love, caring, humor, and continuous support.

Last, but not least, special thanks to Rhodes & Easton and the Jenkins Group, Inc. team, especially Jerry Jenkins, Alex Moore, Theresa Nelson, Mary Jo Zazueta, Anne Stanton, and Eric Norton for helping to make this book a reality.

# Chapter 1

# *F*EEL *THE* *E*MOTIONAL *D*ANCE

*W*hen surgery is suggested, people react differently to the news. With an emergency operation, there may not be time for a strong emotional reaction. But with an elective surgery, the emotional shifts can increase.

Proposed surgery triggers a flood of emotions with most people. Shock, disbelief, anger, frustration, disorganization, fear, anxiety, or sadness can be part of the process. Awareness of this internal turmoil is key; feeling these sensations is powerful to the whole experience. Managing these emotions, over time, helps to ease the surgery and recovery process.

### *Shock Brings Numbness*

For some men and women, the shock of a diagnosis or suspected problem brings about a numbness which protects them temporarily and eases the experience of what is happening. This automatic response, which is quite

miraculous, offers a reprieve from the confusion of handling too many emotions at once. This paralysis also slows
the drain on energy resources, an important savings needed
for surgery.

Some people react with anger, due to the inconven-
ience of the surgery or seriousness of the situation. The
*why me* battle begins as frustration spins out of control.
Why me? Why now? Why do I deserve this?

### *What If's*

The *what if's* march in your head. What if they find
a serious problem? What if I do have cancer? What if I
need more surgery or follow-up treatments? What if I need
more time off of work? What if I can't take care of my
family? What if I can't accept the body changes following
surgery? What if I can't deal with what is happening now?
In the future?

Emotionally, the what if's fuel the fears; anxiety
floods from within. Sadness, bargaining, and acceptance
can arrive. This *grieving* process, often accompanied by
mental disorganization, affects some individuals who realize
that following surgery their body can never be the same.
These emotions shift back and forth, causing confusion.
Emotional healing can take a very *long* time, particularly
when a life threatening disease is found.

### *Relief*

But positive emotions can also occur. People may
feel relieved, even joyful, when they hear a definite diagnosis, realize that a medical crisis can be resolved, or recog-
nize that a chronic problem can be corrected. The antici-

pated resolution of a continuous problem brings a calming effect. It soothes individuals mentally, emotionally, physically, and spiritually.

Four progressive movements help people needing surgery. The acronym L-I-V-E is worth noting.

L = LISTEN to the surge of emotions.
I = IDENTIFY your feelings.
V = VALIDATE their normalcy.
E = EXPERIENCE the feelings.

Accept the fact that emotional turmoil happens to most people facing surgery. Although the number of emotions, kinds of feelings, and intensity may vary, one thing is clear: the feelings need to be confirmed, then experienced.

### *Managing Emotions*

Changing emotions can be managed in several ways over time. Talking to people who have had surgery is helpful; speaking with individuals who have had the same surgery is even better. Finding a self-help group or support group that is relevant to your specific problem can be powerful. To seek reassurance, consult your surgeon or the nursing staff.

### *Sadness*

To deal with sadness, write a journal. Bring the emotions down on paper to clear the mind and ease the emotional intensity. Cry and let the tears flow, because the tears linked to emotions cleanse you. Surround yourself with caring and supportive people. Reach out for professional support from a clergy member, counselor, social worker, therapist, psychologist, or psychiatrist, especially with persistent or intensifying sadness.

### *Nudge Anger*

Some people feel angry and out of control when an unwanted surgery is necessary. Everyone manages this frustration differently. Some people release anger constructively, while others repress it, sliding into a state of denial. Some men and women seethe with anger, rather than express it, until this brewing emotion erupts and causes over-reactions.

Anger can be handled by physical activity or other strategies. Physical exercise diffuses the adrenalin and other stress hormones set off by the emotion, and eliminates these toxic chemicals. Venting with friends, listening to music, writing a journal, or stroking a pet also ease this emotion.

To tranquilize the spirit, you can use mental techniques. Visualization can nudge anger out. When you shower, imagine the anger streaming down your body as the water flows over you. Using your senses and imagination, feel the release of anger as the water washes it away and whirls it down the drain.

In addition, you can release anger by combining visualization with deep breathing. After inhaling and holding your breath momentarily (while scanning your body for anger), you can pucker your lips then blow out the breath while visualizing a red cascade escaping. You can see the anger flowing out your mouth, rushing down your arms and out your fingers, rushing down your legs and out your toes.

Emotions can dance when you are faced with surgery. Give yourself permission to feel them, knowing that in time they can be worked through.

### *Keys for Taking Control:*

✓ Understand the different emotions connected to your surgery.
✓ Allow time to work through them.
✓ Strengthen yourself with mental and physical skills.
✓ Seek professional help if feelings cannot be worked through or the grieving process is prolonged.

\* \* \* \* \*

THE ACTIVITY FOR TODAY:

*IDENTIFY ONE STRONG EMOTION THEN WRITE ABOUT IT.*

\* \* \* \* \*

# Chapter 2

# EXAMINE THE NUTS & BOLTS OF INSURANCE

*W*ith a surgery, everyone knows the importance of choosing the right surgeon. But how does the health insurance plan affect that choice? For most people, their medical benefit package influences who performs the operation, which facility does the procedure, how extensive the surgery will be, how long they will be in the hospital, and what will be financially covered. You will have to *pay* for anything not covered in your insurance plan.

Whether you belong to a Health Maintenance Organization (HMO), Preferred Provider Organization (PPO), Independent Practice Association (IPA), Medicare, Medicaid, or other healthcare group, study the surgical criteria carefully.

Because of soaring healthcare costs, health organizations have been urged to look at expenses. In some ways, this has been needed for a long time. Some healthcare groups have made bold decisions to cut costs, yet experts are now questioning if these cost-cutting measures have compromised the quality of healthcare services.

### *Reality Check*

Do a reality check on your coverage by sorting out the nuts and bolts of your insurance. Before you decide on the surgeon, read your medical benefit package thoroughly. There are severe *financial penalties* for not following the requirements for an operation, especially with an in-patient procedure. With out-patient (same-day) procedures, don't assume there will be full coverage by your healthcare plan.

Some policies cover 100% of the care, but others limit coverage, which is a serious problem with an in-patient procedure. You may find that there is a deductible of $500.00 up to thousands of dollars, or no deductible at all. If there is a deductible, *you* pay.

And that is why some people are investigating *major medical* policies to supplement their standard health insurance policy, since very few people have savings accounts to pay hospital bills.

Some people have several health insurance plans from which to choose. Others have a health insurance policy plus Medicare. Check your benefits carefully.

### *Obtain Help*

Many healthcare plans give you a list of specific physicians (within specialties) to consider for your surgery to obtain the best financial coverage. If you are having out-patient surgery, call the benefit analyst with your insurance company to discuss the surgery and get *documented* approval ahead of time.

If you are having in-patient surgery, talk to the surgeon, the surgeon's nurse scheduling the procedure, the hospital admission's coordinator, as well as the insurance benefit analyst. For additional information, consult your employer and the benefits person within the personnel department at work.

For an in-patient procedure, your case needs to be reviewed before the hospital admission is approved for coverage. Depending upon your diagnosis and type of surgery needed, you will be allowed a certain number of days in the hospital that will be partially or fully reimbursed. Your surgeon receives the information on defined limits in your case, so use this physician as a resource. If you are worried about the coverage for rehabilitation or needed treatments following the operation, clear this up with the insurance company.

Keep a careful *log* of all communications. Write down dates, whom you talk to, the questions, responses, and other information discussed. Request all information in writing and keep a *copy* of every completed form turned in and your communications. Double check everything, especially with an in-patient surgery.

### *Second Opinion?*

Some health insurance plans mandate a second opinion before surgery. If you do not comply, financial coverage can be severely cut. Other insurance plans have found that second opinions are not cost-effective. But even without a mandate, some men and women feel strongly about getting a second opinion. If you seek a second opinion without it being required, your consultation might not be reimbursed and it becomes your *out-of-pocket* expense.

Finding a physician for a second opinion can be done in several ways. First, follow the list of specific physicians within your healthcare group, if this applies. You can search out information on them. Call the state medical society, medical associations, medical schools, university hospitals, other hospitals, or healthcare facilities in your area for recommendations. Document how often the names of the surgeons on your required list come up in a positive way. Your family practice or primary care physician or healthcare provider can also help you make the final decision.

For more information about a surgeon, ask around your community. Talk to nurses and social workers who work in hospitals and health agencies, other healthcare professionals, friends of yours who have had surgery, and self-help or support groups related to your problem.

Sort out the nuts and bolts of your healthcare insurance plan *before* you secure the surgeon, because your medical program governs that choice. Financially, you can't afford to do it any other way.

## *Keys for Taking Control:*

✓ Study the surgical benefit package within your healthcare plan.
✓ Keep a copy of all communications.
✓ Obtain a second opinion if it is mandated by your health plan.
✓ Reach out to community and state resources for information.

\*   \*   \*   \*   \*

### THE ACTIVITY FOR TODAY:

*READ THE BENEFIT PACKAGE FROM YOUR HEALTHCARE INSURANCE PLAN THAT RELATES TO YOUR SUGGESTED SURGERY AND MAKE A LIST OF QUESTIONS THAT NEED EXPLANATION.*

\*   \*   \*   \*   \*

# Chapter 3

# SECURE THE RIGHT SURGEON

$S$ecuring the right surgeon is one of the most important decisions you will make. Perhaps your health problem has been followed by a surgeon for months and the physician/client relationship is positive and solid. Then you are all set. On the other hand, maybe your family doctor found the problem and has referred you to a surgeon. Occasionally, you may need to find your own specialist. If your operation is an emergency procedure, you may not have options.

### *The 3 C's to Quality*
Consider the three C's when choosing your surgeon:
- ► Competence.
- ► Caution.
- ► Characteristics.

*Competence* and experience are number one in importance because your life is on the line. All operations carry risks, no matter how major or minor they are. All surgeons are human; mistakes do happen. Your goal is to reduce risks for surgical complications by choosing the right surgeon within your healthcare insurance plan.

To most people, *credentials* are important. Physicians attend medical school, complete a residency program within a specialty, seek a state license to practice, and become certified within the facilities where they do surgery. In many states, physicians are mandated to get a specific amount of continuing education credits annually.

Some surgeons are nationally board certified; other physicians who perform surgery might be board certified within their specialty but are not board certified in surgery. Although many people insist that their surgeon be board certified in surgery, others may choose a physician, board certified within a specialty, with an outstanding, lengthy surgical record.

A surgeon who is certified by the American Board of Surgery has graduated from an accredited medical school, has completed five years of graduate surgical education in an accredited surgical residency program, and has gone through written and oral examinations along with extensive interviews. To check if a surgeon is board certified, you can call the surgeon's office, The American Board of Medical Specialties, or you can look it up in *The Official American Board of Medical Specialties Directory of Board Certified Medical Specialists.*

### *Experience Counts*
Along with the surgeon's credentials, you can check length of surgical experiences by contacting the State Medi-

cal Society or State Medical Licensing Boards. These agencies control the quality of surgery for public protection. Nationally, the American College of Surgeons and the American Medical Association have watch-dog roles over physicians doing surgeries. Ask healthcare professionals about the experience and reputation of specific surgeons.

### *Facility Accredited?*

Investigate the hospitals or clinics allowed by your insurance plan. Most important, you want a healthcare setting that is *accredited* by the Joint Commission for the Accreditation of Healthcare Organizations and licensed by the state agency. The majority of hospitals are accredited. Interest in patient satisfaction and quality control have peaked nationally. You want a facility that is clean, safe, well-staffed, and has a strong *infection control* program.

For in-patient procedures, people may choose a hospital associated with a university, a specialty hospital, or a hospital close to home for the convenience of family and friends. If people know they will need extensive rehabilitation or treatments following the operation, they may choose a hospital with those treatment opportunities. Costs of healthcare settings differ, so investigate this.

Some surgeons operate in several hospitals so you and the physician can choose the best care for your specific operation. With a same-day surgery, you can investigate surgical clinics for another option.

### *Conservatism is Positive*

*Caution* is an important quality. The surgeon should be a conservative provider: there is *no rush* to schedule the elective surgery and *no push* for radical procedures. An elective operation is a last resort. It is scheduled only after conservative measures have been exhausted, such as prescription drugs, consultation with specialists, physical therapy, hormonal treatments, re-evaluation, and repeated examinations of the problem over time.

### *Mutual Respect*

*Characteristics* to look for in a surgeon are patience, communication skills (especially listening skills), caring, approachability, understanding, sensitivity, willingness to share information, respect for confidentiality, and a positive responsiveness to your questions. You want a physician who will take adequate time to meet your needs and who does not feel threatened by your desire for answers. Defensiveness, abruptness, a patronizing attitude, or failure to respond to your questions are red flags. Consider someone else.

Trust and mutual respect build over time and are necessary for a comfortable relationship. Sometimes, people compromise a few non-critical personal qualities for a competent, experienced surgeon with a more business-like personality. This is a personal choice. Frequently, people interview the surgeon prior to the first appointment.

### *Ask Questions!*

At the first appointment, ask questions of the surgeon, watch the body language, and sense your comfort level while responses are given. Take notes or have a support person with you to write responses down. A tape recorder is another option, but first get permission from the surgeon.

Here are sample questions to ask:

*Why?* Why do I need the surgery? What are the risks? What will happen if I don't have the surgery? Are there other options? What are the chances of success?

*Where?* Is the surgery done on an out-patient or in-patient basis? Which facilities do you use?

*How?* How will you do the surgery? What incisions will be made, where will they be made, and how long will they be? How long will the surgery take?

*Anesthesia?* Are there different types of anesthesia that are used with this surgery? Do I have a choice regarding the type of anesthesia? What are the risks? Can I choose my anesthesiologist?

*After?* What can I expect following the surgery? Will there be pain and how will it be managed? What length of time might I be in the hospital? Will I need help at home? What will my limitations be? How long will I be off work? When can I return to daily activities? When can I resume sexual relations?

*Experience?* How many years have you performed this surgery? How frequently do you perform this operation? What are your credentials?

*Fees?* What are your fees and payment schedules?

These questions help you to gain information on important points. Later, you can decide which issues need further discussion. As you clarify information, you will feel more positive as the discussion progresses or the reverse. Gut level feelings are important, so listen to them.

It's a *plus* if the surgeon takes time with you and uses a model, colorful visuals, diagrams, or drawings to increase your understanding of how the surgery will be done.

Remember that if you are rushed, interrupted, intimidated, or patronized, choose another surgeon. Take your time in making the decision.

Securing the right surgeon is vital to your comfort, safety, and success with the surgery. You want a physician who views you as a partner in a collaborative venture. In the end, *you* hold the power to make the final decision.

---

### *Keys for Taking Control:*

✓ Check out the surgeon's credentials, competence, and experience.
✓ Make sure the surgeon is a conservative healthcare provider.
✓ Assess the physician's positive qualities.
✓ Ask questions about the "why" and "how" of the surgery before making a decision.

---

\* \* \* \* \*

THE ACTIVITY FOR TODAY:

*CIRCLE THE ABOVE QUESTIONS YOU WANT TO ASK THEN WRITE ADDITIONAL ONES.*

\* \* \* \* \*

# Chapter 4

# MANAGE THE ISSUES YOU CAN CONTROL

*Y*ou're going to have surgery; the decision is made. With an emergency surgery, you may feel upset, calm, relieved, or out of control. There is no time to take charge. With an elective surgery, you might feel relieved or vulnerable. If your sense of control falls, your stress level soars, so take charge of the issues within your control.

Grab back some power by choosing to take action. Here are ideas: start a home medical file, seek information, talk to people who have had surgery, use resources, and take responsibility for the physician/client relationship.

Perhaps you started a home medical file years ago. If so, congratulations. But if you do not have one, get started *now*, because a health record helps in several ways:

1. It gives you baseline and on-going information on your medical tests should you develop health problems in the future or there is an emergency and your physician is not available.

2. It offers ease in switching physicians or if records are lost.
3. It provides health information to carry when you travel, especially if you have a chronic disease.
4. It helps you to understand and monitor your health care, which is essential to your wellness.
5. It provides a health history for family members.

In the medical file, you might have copies of physical exams, laboratory and X-ray results, summaries of special tests, physician's notes of explanation, blood pressure readings, consultation summaries, or other medical information. For a more organized system, keep it in chronological order with the most recent health findings on top.

### *Information and Power*

Knowledge is power. Reach out for educational materials because learning strengthens you during this sensitive time. Absorb information through seeing, hearing, and touching. You can view graphics and read material. You can listen to positive descriptions and hear instructions. You can touch and work medical models. Understand the *why* of the operation and *how* the problem can be resolved.

For help, obtain information from your surgeon and the professional staff first. By now, your surgeon has probably described the surgery using drawings, videos, or models. Ask for articles from health journals and magazines relevant to your problem.

The nurse scheduling your surgery is an excellent resource. Request brochures that describe your surgery, autologous blood donations (if applicable), pain management options, and written pre-operative instructions.

Make contact with the hospital or clinic where you are having surgery. Do they have a class for people who are having your operation? Some facilities provide classes for patients and their families; they discuss the operation, give tips for after surgery, and include a helpful question and answer period.

### Consumer Information

Libraries offer a wealth of information, so explore the nearest medical library. If the library is restricted to medical, nursing, and technical literature, take a healthcare professional along to interpret the information.

The consumer information section within medical libraries provides information on surgery, nutrition, cancer, and stress, as well as other health topics. The library staff might help you start a computer search. Some libraries allow the copying of articles without a charge or for a nominal fee.

Even the summaries of articles in recognized medical journals, like the *Journal of the American Medical Association,* can be understood by most lay persons. You can check nursing and other health articles in the *Index Medicus* for the latest topic updates.

Universities with medical or nursing schools may have library resources open to the public. The local cancer society, wellness clinics, or public health departments offer educational materials, too. There are many choices.

### Helpful Groups

For additional information, contact national health groups that relate to your specific problem or health agencies that have a health line or hot-line staffed by nurses or health professionals. Also, self-help groups offer mental, emotional, and physical support with specific health problems. Call your state self-help clearinghouse to get connected with the nearest group to match your need. No one can understand better than people going through the same experience.

In self-help or support group gatherings, men and women offer each other new information, express their fears, share their progress or setbacks, give support to their peers, and *learn* from each other. See the self-help and national resources within the appendices.

### *Surfing*

Surfing the NET (Internet) gives medical information, but be *cautious*; retrieve articles only with reliable references. If you do not have access to the Internet, ask a friend, co-worker, or library staff person to help you. No matter how rare your health problem might be, information can be found. Many national health organizations are on-line with their own web page. Several websites are listed with the national resources appendix.

### *Your Needs*

Taking charge also means being assertive and responsible for your part in the surgeon/client relationship. State your needs clearly. Get your needs met. Be brief, direct, and honest in your questions as well as your answers. Always write down the questions and leave room for responses. Requests, complaints, or problems need to be expressed because your surgeon needs feedback.

As information on your surgery increases, your fears and anxieties will decrease.  By taking charge of those issues within your control, you will feel more comfortable with the surgery.

## *Keys for Taking Control:*

✓ Start a home medical file.
✓ Obtain educational materials from your surgeon and other sources.
✓ Seek support from health groups.
✓ Assert yourself to get needs met.

\* \* \* \* \*

THE ACTIVITY FOR TODAY:

*CALL OR VISIT ONE RESOURCE TO EDUCATE YOURSELF ABOUT THE SURGERY.*

\* \* \* \* \*

# CHRISTINA'S STORY

*"I visualized comfort
coming in and pain
going out."*

**FOLLOWING** surgery, the chemical coma kept me
still for five days. It allowed the swelling in my brain to go
down and my healing process to begin. While my family
visited, they watched the monitors I was connected to for
any physiological response from me. With one monitor, the
needle moved a little when my husband or parents spoke to
me; it went wild when my sons talked to me. Everyone
reminded me continuously how much I was loved and how
concerned everyone was.

Waking up from the coma was confusing because
family members weren't at my bedside and my hands were
tied down to protect me. Anxiety and agitation set in.
When the nurse came into the room, I wanted to talk but I
couldn't because of the tube down my windpipe. I tried to
write but I was unable to do so. Several nurses worried
that I might have brain damage because they could not
grasp what I was attempting to write. I thought they were
trying to keep something from me.

This was the hardest and most frustrating time for me
because of the lost five days, not knowing what had
happened, and not being able to express myself, nor to be

22

*understood. Eventually, as I came out of the drugs, I remembered what had happened.*

*On my son's graduation day, May 31, 1992, a splitting headache, unrelieved by medication, nagged at me all day. Although I didn't feel well, I pushed myself through the activities. While talking to some women at one of the graduation open houses, I suddenly heard a pop in my head. Heat shot quickly across the right side of my head and I felt like I was going to pass out.*

*As I moved outside for fresh air, two boys raced to get my husband. One look at me, and he took me home. After our ambulance friends checked my vital signs, they rushed me to the community hospital. By this time, it hurt to keep my eyes open, and any amount of light was too much to tolerate. My headache worsened; I felt nauseated. After an assessment and some tests, I was transferred immediately to a larger hospital for a CAT scan and further assessment with new physicians.*

*Quite remarkably, fear and panic never gripped me; I sensed that everything would be okay. I didn't know what the outcome would be, but whatever would happen, I knew everything would be all right. A calmness embraced me. Sleepiness was arriving; the pain was intensifying.*

*Refusing to panic, I soothed myself with relaxation techniques. With the throbbing pain of the headache, I visualized ocean waves; comfort coming in and pain going out when the waves receded. Using the heat and the searing pain as a white light, I imagined that the white light was coming in to heal me. By now, I was floating in and out of consciousness.*

*My husband sensed he was losing me and asserted himself with the hospital staff; they weren't moving fast enough. As he sought out the attending physician, the doctor, too, was furious that the CAT scan wasn't done. At that point, my husband pursued hospital personnel, clarified deadlines firmly, and followed-up to get action.*

*When the CAT scan showed a brain hemorrhage, I now became an emergency. Hospital personnel scurried around knowing I needed an immediate neuro-care unit. After contacting four major hospitals, a neuro-surgeon in Lansing, Michigan, facilitated a transfer of another patient to make room for me—what a miracle.*

*The physicians were amazed at me, because according to the CAT scan, I should have been in a coma. Shifting in and out of consciousness, I could answer their questions.*

*During the family conference with my husband, Darwin, our two sons, Damon and Aaron, ages 14 and 18 respectively, and my parents, the neuro-surgeon told us that an aneurysm had burst in my brain, although it had temporarily sealed itself off. He reviewed the options. With surgery, there were risks such as brain damage, paralysis, death, a stroke, or personality change. On the other hand, if I didn't have the surgery, the aneurysm could rupture again at any minute. I turned to my husband and said, "I don't see that there is an option." We all agreed.*

*Explaining further, the surgeon told us he would go into the skull and lift the brain lobe to move through other lobes to the hemorrhage which was in the middle of my brain, near the optic (eye) center. Giving me this information was helpful because I could use the knowledge to create images to help heal myself.*

*From Mickey Mouse and the Great Sorcerer, I chose images of the cistern overflowing and water everywhere. I visualized mops dancing around in the back of my eyeballs sopping up the extra blood that had spilled. Imagery and deep breathing techniques eased the severe pain.*

*Although my family support was very strong, they could only see me once an hour before surgery. Concerned with how this whole ordeal might affect my sons, it was very important to me that my son, Aaron, go through with his graduation open house the following Saturday—no matter what happened. I reviewed the food, the location, and all of the details, everything was in place. Now I could "let go" and have surgery, knowing that Aaron would have his special day. There was an acceptance of what life had given me, no fear.*

*My support was overwhelming. Because of my Native American heritage, my family and friends were sending prayers up in smoke, sweet grass burnt for me. Within their religious practices, my Jewish, Christian, and Hindu friends prayed for me. At the college where I taught, my colleagues were deeply concerned, highly supportive.*

*After extensive preparations and being readied for surgery, my entire family, relatives, and pastor surrounded me. Knowing that everything would be okay, I went into surgery wrapped in a blanket of love and prayers. Whatever my healing would be, even if it meant death as a healing, it would be fine, true acceptance. It was June 2, 1992.*

*Following surgery, my hospital time extended well over three weeks. One day my neuro-surgeon bounced into the room and said, "I have good news and bad news." The good news was that the aneurysm had been successfully clipped and the surgery had been a success. The bad news was that a second aneurysm had been discovered. "Well, SHIT," I said.*

*Thinking about the bad news, I tried to pull some positives. The second aneurysm was much smaller and on top of the upper right lobe so they could use the same incision and remove the same piece of bone to get to the aneurysm. The surgery would be performed in three months, after my brain waves had stabilized and it was safe to do the invasive surgery once again.*

*My neuro-surgeon gave me my restrictions regarding the first surgery. I couldn't drive, shop, do dishes, cook, or anything. Pulling on my sense of humor I asked, "Could I get that in writing?"*

*Returning home, my body dictated what I could and could not do. The fatigue was horrendous. Sometimes after just a bath, a nap was welcoming. Reading was out; my eyes couldn't focus. Watching TV didn't work; the stimulation gave me headaches. There was no physical strength to do anything. I focused completely on healing myself.*

*My Native American background had always helped me to manage life's challenges. As a child, my grandfather had taught me lessons and had given me tools, such as visualization, relaxation techniques, nature, humor, self-healing concepts, and belief in a higher power for guidance and direction in life. Over the years, I had tested all of these strategies; they were powerful. Even though my life appeared to be on a precarious balance, I still made life-giving choices and tried to keep a positive attitude to boost my immune system for healing*

*I sailed through the second surgery and the recovery was much more rapid. Slowly, I resumed teaching with only one class at first. In one year, my only residual problem was left-sided weakness. In two years my medical release arrived, and at three years my recovery seemed complete and energy levels returned. Today, I am managing a full schedule.*

*Through all of these experiences, my message to others is that healing comes in many forms. We have to let* go of control and trust a higher power to take care of the healing, no matter what form that healing takes. It could mean death or possibly a disability. We can't feel guilty for what happens.

From the surgeries, I learned to listen to my inner voice, to quiet the outside world, and to get in touch with my inner self. Now, I don't always have to be in control. I have learned that it's okay to allow other people to do things for me.

Balancing on the edge between life and death was one of life's lessons that was meant to be mine. Everyday there are messages to be learned. We never know if tomorrow we, or our loved ones, will be around. Tomorrow is not a guarantee but a gift. Let's not waste it!

# Chapter 5

# CONSIDER YOUR OWN BLOOD DONATION

*W*hen you go to the hospital or surgical clinic for surgery, you may be asked to sign a consent form to allow public blood transfusions if complications occur. This request, although more common with major operations, is sometimes made with out-patient surgeries if the risk of blood loss exists. Most major hospitals have all blood types on hand or they can obtain them from regional centers.

Today you can also donate your own blood to have on hand for the operation. This is called an autologous blood donation. Giving your own units of blood may be desirable yet this is not always possible. If you are anemic due to iron deficiency or bleeding problems, or are having a surgery that might entail considerable blood loss, you may not be allowed to donate. Recently new research recommended that some women having hysterectomies should not donate their own blood because bleeding problems may increase. Timing is also a concern if the surgery is an emergency or scheduled soon.

If you cannot donate your own blood, you can enlist family members or trusted friends with the same blood qualities to donate blood units for you. Your surgeon needs to know if you have directed donors. Make sure that you understand all of the limitations and requirements of the donations, fees, or additional blood procedures, particularly when blood-related family members donate.

### Safer Blood Transfusions

Some people remain cautious of blood transfusions from public donors despite the fact that the blood supply is safer today than ever before. More precise screening is used and blood testing for AIDS and other diseases has improved over the past decade. According to some experts, the risk of getting the AIDS virus from a blood transfusion is about two in 1 million; the risk of getting hepatitis is greater than AIDS.

### Prescription Needed

If your surgery is scheduled months away, ask now about donating your blood. Your surgeon must write a prescription and indicate how many units of blood might be needed for your specific surgery.

Call the nearest American Red Cross Center and talk to the autologous department. Ask about fees then check your insurance coverage because your surgical benefits *may not cover* the testing, handling, or transportation to and within the hospital unless the units of blood are actually transfused.

### *Donation Process*

If you decide to use your own blood, the blood center will schedule you for the donation. Avoid giving blood close to your surgery date. Generally your blood donations start four to six weeks before surgery. If you are donating two pints of blood, they may be drawn one week apart.

Allow two hours for each donation visit even though it may take less time, and make sure you have a light meal or snack before going to the blood center to reduce problems with lightheadedness or dizziness. The blood center usually offers a small snack and beverage prior to and following the donation.

The staff will ask you about your health history and weight, check your temperature, pulse, and blood pressure, then take a drop of blood to make sure you have adequate red blood cells or hemoglobin to safely donate your blood. Hemoglobin is a substance in the red blood cells that carries oxygen to the body organs and tissues. If everything is fine, one unit of blood will be taken.

When your pint of blood has been obtained, you will wait at the center for a brief time to make sure you are all right. Your blood unit will be labeled with your name, identification number, surgery date, and the name of the facility where you will have surgery. You might receive an identification number for each donated unit to take to the hospital for placement on your chart.

Your blood unit will be carefully tested for blood type and other blood components and screened for problems such as AIDS antibodies, hepatitis viruses, syphilis, and other viruses. Within four workdays or so, your blood will be transported to the hospital. If your surgery is delayed for any reason, contact the Red Cross since your units of blood can sometimes be frozen.

### *Build Up Your Blood*

Each time you donate blood, your red blood cell volume and hemoglobin decrease. You want your blood built back up *prior* to the operation. Therefore, ask your surgeon for guidance regarding a prescription for iron or getting iron supplements over the counter along with increasing your dietary intake of iron rich foods. Read the chapter titled "Rebuild Your Blood" for key information on choosing foods high in iron and taking iron supplements.

Donating your own blood to have on hand the day of surgery is an option to consider. For some people, it is a relief to donate the blood or to choose their own donors.

## *Keys for Taking Control:*

✓ Consider autologous blood donation.
✓ Discuss this option with your surgeon
  and the American Red Cross.
✓ Check your insurance coverage.
✓ Build up your blood if you donate before
  surgery.

\* \* \* \* \*

THE ACTIVITY FOR TODAY:

*WRITE DOWN THE PROS AND CONS OF
DONATING YOUR BLOOD FOR THE SURGERY.
TAKE ACTION IF THIS IS AN OPTION FOR YOU.*

\* \* \* \* \*

# Chapter 6

# *P*UT *Y*OUR *L*IFE *IN* *O*RDER

*H*aving an elective surgery gives you an opportunity to put your life in order. Perhaps you have talked for years about drawing up a medical durable power of attorney or a living will. These advance directives state your instructions regarding health care and treatments. Now is the time to plan these documents, with *legal guidance*, to help you, your family, the healthcare administration, and your physician. It is much better to plan ahead than to wait for a crisis when you are incapacitated and cannot express your wishes.

A medical durable power of attorney designates a person, called an *agent*, to make decisions regarding your medical care if you become incapacitated (determined by several physicians). General powers allow an agent to make more decisions; specific powers limit the agent's authority. This advocate strives to have your healthcare plans and wishes honored.

### Shared Values

When you select an agent, consider several factors. Choose a family member or close friend who lives nearby. Avoid your physician or any person with a vested interest in you, because this could violate the law. Very important, you want an agent whom you can trust and who shares your values on medical treatments and religion. Equally powerful, this advocate must have the ability to be objective, decisive in a crisis, and *courageous* in carrying out your plans. All of these issues need to be discussed thoroughly with the potential agent and a firm commitment needs to be obtained.

Without the power of attorney document, no one has the legal authority to make healthcare decisions for someone else, even a spouse or family members. Today, about two-thirds of states have laws allowing the use of medical power of attorney documents.

### Life Sustaining Treatments?

The second document, a living will, which may not be binding in all states, provides general guidelines (personalized instructions or wishes) on the type of care or extent of treatment you wish to receive. To make it more binding, a living will is sometimes signed in conjunction with a medical durable power of attorney. Some state statutes require the physician to include the living will in the medical record. A release of the physician and healthcare facility from liability for following advance directives is common.

In the event of a terminal illness or irreversible condition (certified by two physicians), your living will comes into play when you are no longer able to communicate what life-sustaining treatments you want or do not want. Some issues deal with cardio-pulmonary resuscitation, use of a respirator or ventilator, medications, or more controversially, feeding tubes and intravenous feedings, to name a few.

Discuss your wishes and get guidance from your physician and lawyer. Without this written directive, your family is *helpless* in either authorizing the use of or withholding life-prolonging procedures.

Both of these advance directives are signed, dated, and witnessed by two or more people (disinterested parties) and notarized to prevent problems. In some states, the adult witnesses cannot be a relative, potential estate beneficiary, legally responsible relative, or the patient's healthcare provider. These documents remain in effect indefinitely unless you revoke them or express limitations by drawing up a new directive and making it clear that it replaces the old one which is destroyed.

### Distribute Directives

All documents should be distributed to your power of attorney agent, lawyer, physician, hospital, family members, and religious advisor as well as carried in your car. If your doctor has reservations about your wishes, consider another physician. Tell family members that if you are admitted to a healthcare facility with a life-threatening problem, they must give the directives immediately to the physician and nurse in charge at that time.

Since 1991, under the Patient Self-Determination Act, most health facilities are required to inform patients about advance directives. This act also requires health facilities to ask patients if a directive has been signed and prohibits discrimination whether directives have been signed or not.

Each state differs in what directives will be recognized. There is *no guarantee* that your written decisions will be carried out, since it will depend upon your state, healthcare setting, medical team, and your family members. In reality, you have the best chance of having your healthcare wishes respected if you live in a state where both advance directives are recognized. If you reside in several states over the year, investigate the differences in advance directives and pursue different documents if necessary.

As soon as possible, get information on your state's advance directives. Ask your attorney, physician, healthcare facilities, local health departments, state medical associations, bar associations, state representatives, offices on aging, or the hospital admission's office for help. A sample directive and updated information are available from the Choice in Dying organization, the American Association of Retired Persons (AARP), libraries, and from the Internet. If you choose to use free guidelines to write your own, be very *cautious* about understanding what the documents say or don't say; an attorney is a better decision.

Many Americans put off completing advance directives because they say they don't have time or cannot deal with issues of disability or death. But it is a good feeling to have your affairs in order. View these documents as priorities, because planning ahead announces your preferences and removes some burden from your family. Although some medical terminology and procedures are controversial at this time, it is far better to make your wishes known.

## *Keys for Taking Control:*

✓ Research your own state regarding advance directives.
✓ Seek legal guidance.
✓ Choose the right agent for the medical durable power of attorney.
✓ Distribute advance directives properly.

\* \* \* \* \*

THE ACTIVITY FOR TODAY:

*MAKE ONE PHONE CALL TO INITIATE A MEDICAL DURABLE POWER OF ATTORNEY OR A LIVING WILL.*

\* \* \* \* \*

# Chapter 7

# PREPARE THE FAMILY FOR YOUR SURGERY

*W*ith an emergency surgery, family members are involved immediately; there is no time to prepare them. With an elective surgery, there are many choices. You can talk to people about the operation as you feel comfortable. Listen to your feelings. Parents worry, no matter what age you are, so consider what details to give them. If you live alone, you might tell your closest friends or a few neighbors.

### *Family Meeting*

For most families, communicating about the operation is helpful. If you have a spouse, significant partner, or children, call a meeting to discuss upcoming changes. If you are upset about the surgery, the children may feel the tension because stress is contagious, no matter how hard you try to shield them. Without giving details, talk about this event to ease the family strain.

If the possibility of cancer exists, the children do not need to know this before the operation. However once the cancer diagnosis is made, you can decide *when* and *how* to tell them. When one family member is experiencing a difficult time, all family members are affected.

Consider the children's ages when giving information. If they are ten years of age or younger, answer their questions simply and support them in expressing themselves. With older children, you can discuss more details and encourage them to talk about their doubts, confusion, or the need for more information.

### *Non-verbal Cues*

Body language speaks loudly, so watch the children's facial expressions, eye contact, gestures, and behavior for changes. Over 90% of what they communicate is through their tone of voice and body language. Signs that might indicate increased anxiety are: withdrawal, nightmares, insomnia, eating problems, physical complaints, unusual aggressiveness, or a regression to a younger behavior. Sadness, crying jags, or increased anger can indicate stress, too. Talking and reassuring the children may help, but family *counseling* is often needed with lingering illnesses.

With any surgery, sharing information helps the family in five ways:

1. It keeps the lines of communication open and conveys value to family members.
2. It encourages the venting of feelings.
3. It buffers family conflicts.
4. It prepares family members for upcoming changes.
5. It promotes cooperation before and after surgery.

### Let Go of Control

When you have surgery, the management of daily activities needs to be turned over to family members. This surrender of control is difficult for some people. Cooperation increases when family members are included in decisions, so ask them to help plan the hospital and recovery time. They can decide *how* home responsibilities will be divided and completed, which is an important learning experience.

Brainstorm other issues with the older children. Let them determine how to get to school, extra-curricular activities, or part-time jobs. Could other families be involved in car pooling the children temporarily? Could relatives or neighbors help out or the teenagers drive themselves and the younger ones to activities?

If all of your children are pre-schoolers, their ability to pitch in is limited. More than likely, you'll need to *hire* help, *ask* for help from a friend, neighbor, relative, or co-worker, *barter* to have the children stay with someone else, or *choose* a quality child-care setting. Plan this ahead of time.

### Family Support

When you need surgery, it helps to have supportive family members. However, in reality this isn't always the case. Some people face not only the challenge of a serious surgery but insensitive and *uncooperative* members which brings unbearable stress to everyone. Having surgery is a lonely experience that is complicated by non-supportive family members, particularly with a cancer diagnosis and lingering treatments. Family therapy or family counseling is crucial.

Preparing family members for the surgery helps in most families because major changes impact members dynamically. Through communication and involvement, tensions can be relieved that ease the surgical process.

### Keys for Taking Control:

✓ Call a family meeting to discuss upcoming changes.
✓ Keep communication lines open to reduce family tension.
✓ Let family members decide how family activities will continue.
✓ Seek family therapy with lingering illnesses.

\*   \*   \*   \*   \*

THE ACTIVITY FOR TODAY:

*LIST TWO STEPS YOU WILL TAKE TO PREPARE THE FAMILY FOR SURGERY.*

\*   \*   \*   \*   \*

Chapter *8*

# *Organize Your Home & Your Life*

*H*aving surgery bestows several gifts: time to STOP, time to PAUSE, and time to CLARIFY VALUES. An operation stops you in your tracks; it awards a chance for you to regroup. But this pause is difficult when home concerns need attention.

People question how routine tasks will get done during the time of surgery and recovery. Single men and women with full custody of their children anguish over this challenge. In some marriages, both husband and wife take responsibility to get chores done, yet in other families, women take the lead. In one recent study, nearly 90% of the women felt responsible for overseeing *all* family activities.

Surgery changes all of that. Having an operation is a *humbling* experience; it transforms a person in full control into a person with limited control. It commands a letting-go process. There is no other choice.

### *Plan Meals*

With an elective surgery, organizing yourself ahead of time is possible; it eases worries, prevents guilt, and reduces stress. Food, staples, home responsibilities, correspondence, time off, and your support system can be considered in advance.

Many families feel passionate about providing healthy meals for their members, yet this is challenging following a major operation. Some people have help upon returning home, others do not. Even with a same-day surgery, the novelty of getting meals wears off quickly if you feel nauseated, weak, or light-headed.

To relieve this pressure, get family members involved. Have them list quick, easy, and healthy meals for several weeks following surgery. Post their choices on the refrigerator.

Some meals, soups, and sauces can be cooked and frozen ahead of time, such as spaghetti or taco sauce, barbecue, or casserole dishes. Consider that one or two meals each week can be take-out meals. You deserve it.

If desired, you can put pizzas, healthy frozen dinners, breads, juices, lean meats, poultry, fish, and frozen vegetables in the freezer. Choose other meals requiring five to ten minutes of preparation time for family members: scrambled eggs, French toast, or tuna melts. Remember that friends or relatives might bring meals over. Ask for help.

Several days before surgery, stock the refrigerator with fruit, vegetables, eggs, milk, low-fat cheeses, and margarine. A good supply of cereals, crackers, and juices is also helpful.

### Stock Supplies

Staples can be stocked ahead of time, so little by little, buy a six-week supply of items.    Paper products, shaving items, toothpaste, cosmetics, deodorant, shampoo, skin lotion, soaps, detergents, and contact lens products are all helpful to have on hand.    If you have pets, purchase food, treats, and cat litter.

### Straighten the House

Prior to the operation, straighten your home.    Release any compulsion to have a *perfect* house.    Family members can help with the cleaning over a two-week period of time, completing one or two rooms per day.    If family members are uncooperative, you live alone, or work full-time outside the home, arrange for a cleaning person to come in the week before surgery and periodically following the operation for a few months.    No housecleaning is permitted within 48 hours of the procedure.    You don't want to go into surgery exhausted.

### Arrange Jobs

Think ahead about the payment of bills or correspondence and other needs.    Ask a trusted family member, relative, or close friend to oversee bill payments for the first month after a major operation.    If hospital bills arrive, they will need a careful review; reach out to a healthcare professional friend for interpretation.

In addition, birthday, anniversary, get-well, and sympathy cards are helpful to have on hand.    Address and stamp those cards needed over the next two months, then place them in sequence to be mailed.

Other chores can be considered, especially if you live alone. Yard work will need attention; a high school neighbor can be hired to cut the grass or shovel the snow. Also, you'll need people to bring in the mail and newspaper, feed the pet, oversee the litter box, or walk the dog.

## Work Arrangements

For some men and women, organizing your life means planning time off from work, often discussed when surgery is suggested. For some employees, the 1993 Family and Medical Leave Act is an option. Briefly, this federal act requires employers to allow an employee up to 12 weeks of *unpaid* leave during any one-year period of time when a serious health condition affects the employee or a family member. To see if you qualify, talk to your employer or staff member in the personnel or benefits department and get a booklet on medical leave.

## Support Network

For many people, it's helpful to talk about the upcoming operation. To request support, contact your priest, rabbi, or minister, and write or call selected friends and relatives to let them know your surgery date. Ask for thoughts and prayers from them and request that you be added to the prayer list in their church or synagogue. A good support network buffers stress and anxiety; it is important throughout surgery and recovery.

If desired, you might tell the support people that you won't be receiving visitors at the hospital because the stay will be too short, but that your answering machine will be on following surgery and you welcome their get-well messages or cards. Remember that you can call anyone at anytime or request visitors if you feel up to it. Good friends will respect your wishes.

To help the healing process, go through your calendar and *cancel* all commitments throughout the recovery time. You want to be *appointment free* perhaps for the first time in your life.

Make a short list of individuals who have expressed the deepest concern regarding your operation. Post their names and phone numbers, then ask a family member or friend to call them with a progress report after surgery. Take the phone numbers of your three closest friends to the hospital to call if you feel up to it. Stay free of promises; there are always options.

Planning ahead is priceless. Responsibilities need to be released so that energy can be channeled into the operation and healing process.

## *Keys for Taking Control:*

✓ Plan meals and stock up on staples
   before surgery.
✓ Turn over home responsibilities to other
   people.
✓ Review the Family and Medical Leave
   Act.
✓ Secure your support system.

\* \* \* \* \*

THE ACTIVITY FOR TODAY:

*TAKE YOUR CALENDAR AND CANCEL ALL
COMMITMENTS THROUGH THE
RECOVERY TIME.*

\* \* \* \* \*

# Ken's Story

*"My advice to patients is: if you have questions, make sure you get answers; if you disagree, say so."*

*1977.  Two significant events had just happened in my life.  My father had just died.  My son, Jared, had been born and was less than a year old.  While in my doctor's office for a persistent sore throat, he noticed that a light spot on my forehead had changed color.  Within minutes, three physicians surrounded me.  They all agreed that the skin area needed to be biopsied.*

*The biopsy report confirmed a cancer, a basal cell carcinoma.  Since the cream to destroy remaining cancerous cells was ineffective, I was referred to a plastic surgeon for more extensive surgery.*

*Having the word cancer connected to my name was frightening because the word cancer had always meant death.  After all, I wasn't supposed to get cancer because my relatives died from heart problems.  To prevent dwelling on the news, I kept myself busy.*

*I loved my job, working in sales for a national athletic knitwear manufacturer, and enjoyed traveling Michigan to sell the knitwear.  Working on a commission was fine with me, because I was good at sales and provided*

48

*well for my family. From the company president on down, the administration treated each employee as a family member; they couldn't do enough for me once they heard about my health problem.*

*While the plastic surgeon removed the stitches from my extensive skin surgery, I casually asked him about a spot on the back of my left shoulder. His reaction rang a serious note. Within one hour, I was in surgery again, having the mole removed, which was diagnosed as a malignant melanoma, Level III.*

*Since the word melanoma meant nothing to me, I researched the problem at the nearest medical library. I learned that it was the most fatal kind of skin cancer and that my chance of living five years was less than 20%. This was not good news.*

*Because of his young age, my son could not understand what was happening. My wife, Lynne, tried hard to cope with what was happening to me and our family, but she was having a difficult time; everything was happening too fast.*

*My physician referred me to a cancer center out East for a consultation, and carefully prepared, then sent my records. But when I arrived, the professionals didn't know why I was there and had no records on me. This upset me. I walked out of the facility and vowed never to return. My home physician eventually understood my actions and said he would've done the same thing.*

*One morning in 1978, I noticed a lump on the left side of my neck that I suspected could mean more trouble. My physician was equally concerned. The surgery, a radical neck dissection, was extensive. Lymph nodes and tissue were removed, then skin grafting was done at the same time; some of the lymph nodes proved to be malignant.*

*This time my physician insisted that I go for a cancer consultation. After great deliberation, I agreed to try a cancer and tumor institute in Texas. What a welcome I received. This institute cared about people and had a devoted staff that educated me about cancer for the first time. They were honest in answering my endless questions. From the moment I walked into the institute, I was embraced by a warm and caring environment.*

*They wanted me to be a part of their team. After they reviewed all experimental programs open to my specific case, they allowed me to choose the treatment program I wanted. I chose to have immunotherapy that would be followed by chemotherapy. I was given three years to live.*

*Because of my stubbornness, I felt that I would go through the treatments without any serious problems, but the first dose of immunotherapy caused a soaring fever, peaking at 106 degrees, and violent chills. Terror gripped me when I couldn't reach my treatment physician. Later it was suggested that I may have been given the wrong dose.*

*I learned a valuable lesson from that experience. Now, I encourage other people to understand their treatments, get information on possible side effects, and know who to call if something does go wrong.*

*Bluish black spots appeared on my body, one at a time, on a 90-day cycle. One by one they were surgically removed, and the pathology report stated "metastatic malignant melanoma." I was placed on a tuberculosis vaccine. My home physicians explained that these spots meant that my malignant melanoma had spread, and if the spots came increasingly more frequently, I could die.*

*All of the surgeries and the cancer recurrences brought challenges to my family as well as to myself. Relationships were strained. I couldn't discuss everything that was happening with Lynne, which bothered me. Over time, I found that giving my medical updates upset her too much and made things worse, so I kept some things to myself. The physicians suggested professional help for the two of us, but we had difficulty finding the right person. Lynne and I had different concerns.*

*My concerns centered around not just staying alive, but having a quality of life to the end. Financially, I worried about supporting my family, being a role model for my son, and contributing to society. My main goal was staying alive without drowning in self-pity.*

*Lynne feared losing me, being alone, handling the family finances, and having total responsibility for our son. Those fears were real. The stability and security that my wife and son needed the most, I could not give them.*

*My mood wasn't up all of the time. When I felt depressed, it was usually connected to my son. When I thought about him, I would feel bad that I wouldn't see him grow up. Sometimes I felt jerked around like a puppet by circumstances beyond my control.*

*Exercise helped me mentally as well as physically; it was a great release for my frustration and anger. I threw myself into more walking, swimming, weight machines, and jogging. Occasionally at the athletic club, people would give me strange looks because of my surgical scars, but over time I learned to accept my body the way it was.*

*Libraries became my haven. One day, I found a fascinating book lying around called* Death: The Final Stage of Growth *by Elizabeth Kubler-Ross. The book helped me to get in touch with my feelings and experiences; it had me so spellbound that I searched out her other books to read. They touched me deeply because I could relate to them.*

*In 1981, a strange thing happened. A lymph node behind my right ear enlarged, continued to enlarge for about a week, then stopped growing. I waited for weeks and it never budged. Eventually I showed it to my surgeon who removed it, and as he examined it, there was no doubt in his mind that it was related to the malignant melanoma. The pathology report stated that even though the node had all of the ingredients of a malignant melanoma, it was really dead tissue. My doctor told me that whatever I was doing, I should keep it up.*

*This incident got my mind thinking. Does the body have the power to kill a cancer? Can the immune system fight off a cancerous growth? Can the mind help to heal the body? I questioned if people could mentally activate their body's defenses.*

*My monthly tests remained clear for a year. Then in 1982, nagging stomach pains hit me. This was discouraging. Extensive tests revealed tumors in the stomach, right lung, and my liver. Biopsy reports stated metastatic melanoma. I was shocked with the spread of my cancer.*

*In Texas, my physicians agreed about the progression of my disease; they suggested that I get my life in order. But to me, it didn't make any sense that I was dying, because physically I felt pretty good. My gut told me I wasn't dying, which made me more determined than ever to fight the disease.*

*I needed space. I needed time to think about what I was going to do, so I escaped to a university campus nearby and just enjoyed the natural beauty of the area. Returning to the hospital, I talked with my favorite nurse and we shared a laugh. She said she was sorry about what was happening to me, told me to keep up the fight, and reminded me to keep a positive attitude.*

*Returning home, I started to make arrangements. My rabbi and cantor helped me make the funeral arrangements, and I had to laugh because I was getting a 10% discount for thinking ahead with my funeral. My next stop was with my attorney to write up a will and set up a trust for my wife and son, so they would be well provided for. After completing both of these tasks, I felt better about everything.*

*The physicians were more concerned with the tumors in my right lung that were causing me shortness of breath, so they recommended radiation to shrink the tumors before the lung collapsed. Although I initially turned it down, I chose to try the radiation one day at a time. I survived. I turned down more chemotherapy but chose immunotherapy for several months to fight the cancer.*

*My home physician wanted me to see a local oncologist (cancer specialist) and I agreed. I talked with the physician freely about pain control during my illness and to the end. My fear of dying was nothing compared to my fear of getting there. The world lifted from my shoulders as I was guaranteed that my last few months alive would be relatively pain free. Now I could put my energy into living.*

*Fears hit me. I feared that the insurance company would put pressure on my company to discontinue their support to me and my family, so I pushed myself harder at work and produced more than ever before. But my company stood by me 100%. At one national meeting, the sales manager assured me that no matter what happened, I would have my job for as long as I wanted it. What a boost that gave me.*

*At the company headquarters in Rochester, New York, I reviewed retirement benefits. From a logical viewpoint, the best option for my family was for me to retire, but emotionally, retiring was the last thing I wanted to do. By the end of the day, retirement papers had been drawn up. I retired at age 40.*

*Retirement was hard on me because I had been a strong, competitive, hard worker who had been highly productive and successful. That was all disappearing and there wasn't a thing I could do. For a long time I struggled with a loss of identity and self-worth.*

*Guilt also hit. I felt guilty for not working, guilty for being on disability, guilty for being on social security, guilty for being on Medicare, and guilty for being alive. I questioned why I was still living.*

*One month later, four bluish black spots remained on my body, but within three weeks, all of them had disappeared. This was remarkable. Extensive follow-up tests showed no detectable cancer anywhere in my body.*

*I'll never know if the many surgeries, treatments, myself, or divine intervention played a part in my progress, but perhaps it was all four. I also had an attitude that "I will not be defeated," and a tremendous "contempt for the cancer" within me that could've helped me.*

*Over the past 14 years, more surgeries have been required, some serious, some not so serious. Although I was terrified of my first surgery, I am now at ease with the surgical process. If the surgery is done under a local anesthetic, my surgeon and I joke around to pass the time. We have developed a very special relationship over the years.*

*Throughout all of this, I have tried hard to keep a sense of humor. Many times what was happening to me wasn't funny at all. But now looking back, I have been able to chuckle over some episodes along the way.*

*Now, I have both a medical durable power of attorney and a living will drawn up, and periodically, I re-distribute*

*the directives to the right people. My wishes are abundant-
ly known. Cancer patients need the security of knowing
that their wishes will be respected so that their energy can
be directed into their treatments. By taking control of their
lives, they can live a better life.*

*Exercise, especially bike riding, home projects, and
being a house-husband fill part of my life. When possible,
I take college courses and speak with groups, schools, and
organizations on motivational topics. My energy is also
directed into lobbying for national issues I believe in.*

*The cancer and tumor institute in Texas refers
patients with melanoma to me and my medical story is now
on the Internet. On a weekly basis, I hear from people all
over the world and respond to their questions. Most major
hospitals have a referral service for specific cancers and
problems. By helping people, I feel productive.*

*Most of all, I miss working and earning a salary.
Because I cannot risk losing medical benefits for my family,
I can never work again, but now I know how lucky I was
to have worked for a company that cared so much for their
employees.*

*For any surgery, information is the key to success; it
is the most powerful weapon a patient can have. Ignorance
is the enemy. Patients must become knowledgeable of what
is happening to them, take an active role in their health
care, stand up for themselves, and be their own best
advocate. They should never underestimate the healing
ability of their mind and should always remember that they
are the most important member on the medical team.*

*My advice is: if you have questions, make sure you
get answers; if you don't understand something, ask for
clarification; if you have ideas about your case, express
them; if you hear of new treatments, ask your physician to*

*research them; if you disagree with your physician, say so. The best thing a cancer patient can do is to talk to another lay person who has walked through the same experience.*

*The one common thread in people's lives that makes them survivors with a health problem is the fact that they believe that what they are doing is right. I am a firm believer that a patient must believe in the treatment they are getting for it to work.*

*Men and women need to know that they are not alone, that there are other people going through difficult times who are aware of the mental and physical pain that they are feeling. All patients need to sense that they are in control over some things and that what they feel is important. I trust my instincts.*

Reference: Shapiro, Kenneth. *Dying and Living: One Man's Life With Cancer*. Austin, TX: University of Texas Press, 1985.

# Chapter *9*

# *GET PREPARED MENTALLY*

*W*hen emergency surgeries arise, some people lack the time to prepare themselves for the procedure. But with an elective surgery, men and women can help themselves in many ways. Having a positive frame of mind going into an operation improves the *success rate* of the surgery. This attitude also promotes the healing process and helps you return to a healthy state.

### *Your Creative Brain*

With surgery, fears tease the mind, play games with your thoughts, and create rational and irrational images in your head. Rational fears are connected to the unknowns with the surgery. What will the surgeon find? How will the operation change me?

But with irrational fears, your mind exaggerates a simple concern because the imagination knows no bounds. The longer you dwell on the idea, the more it *magnifies* the fear; a vicious cycle evolves. High prices are paid for these distortions: loss of sleep, loss of time, loss of energy, and loss of health.

This vicious cycle creates mental symptoms, such as confusion, indecisiveness, inability to concentrate, or increased anxiety. But you can ease this turmoil and condition the mind for surgery through the following techniques:

- ► Problem-solving.
- ► Shifting your thought pattern.
- ► Scheduling a worry time.
- ► Mentally rehearsing the event.

### Let Go

Problem-solving lowers apprehensions. This exercise can be done in the following steps: document, determine control level, brainstorm, and release.

Start with one issue that is bothering you about the surgery; write it down. Once a problem becomes black and white, you can deal with it. Ask yourself if this concern is *within* your control or *beyond* your control. If the worry is within your control, brainstorm then write steps to take charge of the situation.

Rank the action steps in sequence. For example, you might seek more medical information on your specific problem. Make a commitment to take action rather than let stress immobilize you.

If the problem is out of your control, document how to *release it*. Could you use resources, get professional help, let-go, or give your burden to a higher power? With any written plan, pressure disappears. As you guide your mind through a step-by-step process, confusion melts away and your thought pattern re-organizes itself.

### *Change Your Thought Pattern*

Shifting your thought pattern alters your mental state. This is done by diverting the mind or changing your internal dialogue (self-talk). If you say continuously, "I'll never get through this operation" or "I can't take the pressure of this upcoming surgery anymore," a negative frame of mind develops. This attitude sets up doubts and uncertainties regarding the procedure, which can be unhealthy.

But you can intercept negativity by changing what you say to yourself. Inserting constructive phrases is more helpful. Try saying:

"I will keep a hopeful frame of mind."

"I refuse to let this surgery get me down."

"I know this operation is needed; I'll be okay."

Repeat these soothing phrases over and over; they reassure you. Changing your dialogue is not meant to replace mood fluctuations that happen to everyone facing surgery, but a better frame of mind eases the experience.

Diverting the mind also shifts your thinking. This can be done in many ways: listening to music, exercising, reading, watching TV, working on a craft, or writing a journal. As you focus on something else, your thought pattern changes.

### *Time Your Worries*

For some people, scheduling a worry time calms concerns. This technique allows 30 minutes a day to address your fears. After setting a timer for this interval, you entertain your worries and brainstorm productive outcomes. Focusing on the problems for a limited period of time or creating a worst case scenario is helpful.  Beyond the 30 minutes, dwelling on worries is *not allowed* throughout the day or night.

### *Rehearse the Experience*

Mentally rehearsing the event is a powerful strategy to prepare your mind for surgery.  With this skill, you imagine parts of the surgical experience in a positive way, then repeat this imagery day after day.  For example, you might visualize yourself as strong, healthy, and confident going into surgery or imagine yourself healing more readily following surgery.   Practicing this mental rehearsal for weeks before the operation empowers you and increases a sense of control.

Fears and worries are common when surgery is needed, yet they can sabotage you at this delicate time. Mental strategies hold great power because it is your mind-set that *drives* your physical and physiological responses to the surgery.

## *Keys for Taking Control:*

✓ Problem-solve issues within your control.
✓ Shift your thought process if it is counter-productive.
✓ Set a worry time.
✓ Mentally rehearse a positive experience with your surgery.

\* \* \* \* \*

THE ACTIVITY FOR TODAY:

*PRACTICE ONE MENTAL TECHNIQUE TO PREPARE YOURSELF FOR THE OPERATION.*

\* \* \* \* \*

# Chapter 10

# NOURISH YOUR BODY IN PREPARATION

*I*t's never too late to physically prepare yourself for surgery. Even with an urgent procedure, you can make choices to influence positive outcomes. You want your body to be strong and healthy to prevent problems, speed healing, and aid recovery. Your nutritional state and over-all health impact surgical outcomes.

### *Assess Diet*

For days, weeks, or months before the operation, you can improve upon your self-care. Good nutrition is impor-tant. Resist missing meals, because you need all of the nutrients you can get. Eating right helps your mood, health, energy level, and ability to function in a positive way.

Grazing is in. You might try eating six small meals a day or three small meals and three snacks. This frequency of smaller amounts is gentler on your digestive tract; it also stabilizes your blood sugar and provides on-going energy levels. Snacks might include raw vegetables, a bagel, low-sodium pretzels, low sugar yogurt, or a piece of fruit.

Cut down on your sugar, especially if you crave it. Some experts believe that excessive refined sugar *lowers* your immune system. One study shows that with heavy sugar intake, your body has a 50% *decreased ability* of the white blood cells to destroy bacteria. For surgery, a strong immune system is important. Although you need glucose for brain and body function, you get plenty of that within a healthy diet.

Refined sugar overload can also lower essential nutrients, such as the Vitamin B-complex and a mineral called chromium. The B vitamins soothe your emotions and nervous system, so decreased amounts increase irritability and general nervousness at a time when you are already vulnerable. Chromium helps to *stabilize* your blood sugar levels, so all of these nutrients are important to you.

If you choose to switch from large amounts of sugar to excessive use of sweeteners, be careful with this substitution because some sweeteners have recorded side effects. It may be better to cut back amounts of both of these.

## Caffeine Effects

With surgery, your caffeine intake also needs to be reviewed. This drug stimulates the release of stress hormones, such as adrenalin and cortisol, and heightens anxiety and nervousness. It can cause palpitations (racing heart) and an irregular heart rhythm which could be a problem. Since caffeine can stay in your system eight or more hours, it can rob you of needed sleep or reduce the *quality* of sleep before the operation. You don't need any of these problems.

Because of its addictive qualities, cut back on caffeine *slowly* over several weeks. The latest research has indicated that the headache following many surgeries is nothing more than a caffeine withdrawal reaction.

### Prime the Body

Increasing your water intake to eight glasses per day primes your body for a more successful outcome of the surgery. Water flushes out the kidneys, prevents bladder infections, and eases constipation problems. Since carbonated beverages tax the kidneys, consider cutting down on amounts.

Before some surgeries, increasing dietary fiber lessens problems, too. Adding more fruits, vegetables, and whole grains prevents constipation problems. Before, during, and after surgery, constipation may be caused by medications and the decreased mobility following the procedure.

### Nutrients Are Key

Some vitamins and minerals are essential to surgical outcomes. They promote healing, *boost* your immune system, build up the blood, or replenish depletions caused by stress. Vitamin A aids the repair of body tissue, and Vitamin C heals wounds, forms red blood cells, and fights infections. Under the stress of surgery, Vitamin C can be depleted and increased amounts are necessary, especially for smokers who have a lower blood level of this vitamin.

The Vitamin B-complex provides energy to the body, helps normal functioning of the nervous system, and boosts the immune system. It too must be replenished under stressful conditions. Zinc helps the *healing* process. Iron is crucial to hemoglobin, the oxygen transporter in your bloodstream. Vitamin K is necessary for blood clotting function and calcium helps to regulate the heart beat, is a natural tranquilizer, and together with phosphorous maintains bone strength. All of these nutrients are relevant to surgical success.

First, get these vitamins and minerals from your diet. Fruits and vegetables (especially yellow, orange, and green leafy), fortified low-fat milk, low-fat dairy products, fortified cereals, whole grain enriched breads, beans, seeds, chicken, and fish are only a few examples of healthy foods to eat prior to surgery.

If you do decide to take a supplement, choose a 100% RDA (Recommended Dietary Allowance) multiple vitamin and mineral and take it with food. An increase of water soluble vitamins such as Vitamin C or the B-complex can be considered, but *hold back* from taking any excess of fat-soluble vitamins such as A, D, E, and K or the mineral Zinc because of potential toxicity. Check this out with your surgeon, nutritionist, or a registered dietician. Read the chapter on building up your blood if you give autologous blood donations or are on iron therapy.

One or two weeks before surgery, it is often recommended that you *stop* taking aspirin and Vitamin E since both of these affect your blood clotting process. It's helpful to stop smoking or greatly cut back for two or more weeks before surgery. The drugs in cigarettes constrict your blood vessels, impair circulation, prevent the hemoglobin from carrying oxygen throughout the body, lower the

immune system, and *increase* the chance for infections following surgery, especially pneumonia.

### Increase ZZZZZs

Sleep renews your immune system and replenishes
your energy levels, so try to improve your quality of sleep.
Sleep also *activates* natural killer (NK) cells, a type of
lymphocyte in the blood that helps you resist and fight viral
infections. If you can't sleep, use music, reading, relaxation tapes, a warm bath, or mental techniques to induce
relaxation.

### Walk Away Problems

If possible, increase physical exercise before surgery
because it boosts your oxygen uptake, improves circulation,
activates your *immune* system, and diminishes constipation
problems. Equally impressive, physical activity heightens
self-confidence and self-image; it releases fear, stress,
anger, sadness, and anxiety. Even a 15-minute brisk walk
four times weekly energizes you. Exercise also improves
sleep, benefits your circulation and body systems, and gets
you in shape for the operation.

### Magical Breathing

Deep breathing brings mental, emotional, and physical
benefits; it also helps you to manage the surgical process
better. After a major surgery, the surgical staff will coach
you to use breathing exercises to prevent complications.
For now, inhaling deeply through the nostrils, holding the
breath momentarily, then puckering your lips and *slowly*
blowing out the breath is a start.

Your choices can groom you for a safer and more successful surgical outcome. Nourishing your body in preparation of this event helps with the operation itself, as well as the healing and recovery process.

## *Keys for Taking Control:*

✓ Make dietary choices to reduce surgical problems.
✓ Increase sleep and rest prior to surgery.
✓ Boost surgical success through exercise.
✓ Breathe deeply to practice for the operation.

\*   \*   \*   \*   \*

THE ACTIVITY FOR TODAY:

*WALK FIFTEEN MINUTES TODAY THEN SCAN YOUR BODY FOR ITS POSITIVE EFFECTS.*

\*   \*   \*   \*   \*

# MAKE THE PRE-OP VISIT COUNT

**D**uring this pre-operative visit at the hospital or surgical clinic, you will receive information and get questions answered. Write down specific concerns and bring relevant information from your home medical file, such as current medications, allergies, illnesses, and a list of past surgeries with their dates. Your insurance card(s), blood donation slips, and advance healthcare directives are also important.

This appointment is often completed the week or so before surgery and involves several parts: nurse interview, response to concerns, pre-operative instructions, baseline measurements (blood pressure and other assessments), laboratory, X-ray, and additional testing as ordered by your surgeon or the facility. In some instances, the anesthesiologist's or nurse anesthetist's visit is combined with this appointment, but more likely it occurs on the day of the operation.

## Give and Get Information

During the one-on-one interview with the nurse, your health and family medical history will be reviewed and updated. If you have a chronic disease, such as heart disease or asthma, or are currently suffering from an acute infection, mention this important fact.

Your dental history and injuries from accidents are also important. For example, do you have gold crowns in your mouth, loose teeth, or dentures? Have you sustained neck injuries in accidents or do you have arthritis, especially in the neck? To what degree? All of these questions are relevant to a surgery which requires the insertion of a tube (endotracheal tube) to help your breathing.

## Drug History/Allergies

To prevent complications, your drug history is crucial. Now is the time to tell about drug allergies or sensitivities, side effects to certain medications, or a bad reaction to a certain anesthesia. Listing problem drugs by name is helpful because the nurse can highlight them in your chart, increasing the *safety factor* with your surgery. Mention pain medications that have been effective for you as well as ones that haven't worked. Food and other allergies, such as a latex allergy, also should be discussed. If you had problems with former surgeries, elaborate on them.

## More Information

Give any paperwork that you brought in to the nurse. This might include: abnormal test results, a durable power of attorney for health care, a living will, or autologous blood donation identification numbers, if applicable. If you consulted a specialist, bring the report with you. The nurse might put this information on the chart or request some items for the day of surgery.

During this visit, the nurse will obtain your religious affiliation, names and phone numbers of clergy, and names of people you want contacted in an emergency. Sometimes the consent form for the surgery is signed; sometimes it is held back for the day of surgery. If the form is written in medical terminology, have the nurse write out the operation in lay language above the medical wording, then explain it. Sign the form when you understand *fully* what it says.

Written and verbal pre-operative instructions will be given to guide you in the surgical preparation. They might include dietary changes, when to stop all food and liquids, and what procedures to complete before the surgery. These instructions vary with each procedure.

### *Review the Day*

Before you leave the nurse, get your remaining questions answered and ask for a step-by-step review of the day of surgery. Find out where you should start with the admitting process and ask if you could you have a tour of the surgical area.

Following the interview, measurements and testing are often done, depending upon your surgeon's orders for the same-day or in-patient surgery. Measurements might include: weight, height, pulse rate, blood pressure, and blood oxygen level. Laboratory, X-ray, and additional tests often follow as needed.

Testing varies at each health facility and with each surgery. The hospital or clinic may schedule tests either on-site or off-site. For an out-patient procedure, a Complete Blood Count (CBC) and Chemistry Profile might be ordered, but if there is a chance of bleeding problems, other tests will be required. With a major surgery, you could have all of the above tests plus Blood Type and Screen, Prothrombin Time (blood clotting check), urinalysis, and other laboratory tests.

A chest X-ray, Electrocardiogram (ECG), Echo-cardiogram, Stress Test (treadmill), and other screening tests could be obtained, depending upon your age, family history, symptoms, and medical history.

### Billing Department

Before you leave, make one more stop. Go to the billing department, verify your insurance carrier, and ask that all bills go directly to your insurance company. Upon returning home, you don't want bills arriving. All of your energy must be directed into the recovery process.

Remember that all health facilities manage this pre-operative visit differently. As you obtain more information, your comfort level with the surgery will increase.

## Keys for Taking Control:

✓  Expect resolution of your questions and
   concerns.
✓  Obtain clear pre-operative instructions.
✓  Ask to have the day of surgery reviewed.
✓  Clarify insurance coverage with the
   billing department.

\* \* \* \* \*

THE ACTIVITY FOR TODAY:

*WRITE DOWN THREE QUESTIONS TO ASK
DURING THE PRE-OPERATIVE APPOINTMENT.*

\* \* \* \* \*

# Chapter 12

# CLARIFY ISSUES WITH YOUR SURGEON

*Y*our final appointment with the surgeon is equally important for you and the physician. Frequently, this meeting occurs within one week of the operation and offers a chance to settle remaining concerns.

### Update Information

When you arrive at the office, update your medical history. Focus on your personal, family, and drug/allergy health history. Add to or correct the information, then write the current date with your initials alongside the additions. Copies of these facts go to the hospital or surgical clinic.

Be prepared for this visit. Have a written list of concerns to discuss, leaving a space to write answers. Don't depend upon remembering questions or answers because nervousness can increase at this time, affecting your memory and concentration; it also causes confusion.

73

You might take a support person into the exam room (with permission) to be your ears and to write responses down.

Cluster your concerns around specific topics: the surgery itself, the anesthesia, review of risks, pain control, expectations following surgery, restrictions at home, your information, and final questions. If you can describe what surgery is being done, how it will be accomplished, and what risks there are, this shows a greater understanding of the upcoming operation. The surgeon can add to the description, use a visual aid, or draw out the procedure, which further helps comprehension.

### Issues of Concern

Discuss pain control. What discomfort can you expect and what *options* will be available to you? The physician might ask if you want the Patient Controlled Analgesia (PCA), an intravenous device or traditional injection/oral medications for pain. At this time, talk about your drug tolerance level. How do you handle medications? Your weight is a consideration because the lower your weight, the greater the impact from the drugs. If you rarely take medications, the drugs could impact you more.

Remind your surgeon of other necessary information. If you have a medical durable power of attorney and/or living will, does the surgeon have a copy? If you have given autologous blood donations, mention this. If you have drug allergies/sensitivities or react badly to a specific anesthesia, review the names. Give the surgeon a list of your prescription drugs, then clarify if you have a current infection, a chronic disease, or a health condition requiring antibiotics prior to the procedure.

### *Clarify, Clarify, Clarify*

Express any worries and discuss any questions you have. Be sure to talk about the following:

1. Should you take your prescription drugs the day of surgery? Can you bring medications to the hospital?
2. Can you choose your anesthesiologist? Are there different types of anesthesia used with your operation and do you have choices?
3. How long will the surgery take? How long will you be in the recovery room? Will you wake up with any tubes or catheters inserted or any other aids?
4. What can you expect following surgery? How long will you be hospitalized?
5. Will you need assistance at home? What will be your limitations? How long will it take before you return to daily activities and work?
6. Will there be follow-up treatments or rehabilitation commitments?

Some of the questions cannot be answered until after the operation, yet many answers are necessary, not only for you but for your family members or support people. For example, if assistance is needed at home or special equipment is required, arrangements can be made ahead of time. This is beneficial since hospital stays are brief and most preparations are necessary before returning home.

### *Brief Exam*

The physician might re-examine the area where surgery will take place, then do a brief physical exam, including a check of your heart and lungs for problems. If you are over 40, depending on your family and personal health history, you might have an ECG, additional heart or lung work-up, or other testing to rule out problems. Your surgeon will also gather needed information.

This vital appointment helps you and your surgeon, because the giving and receiving of information is essential to surgical success. Be assertive to get your questions and concerns responded to. Remember the 5 W's: who, what, where, when, and why. Knowledge calms apprehensions with the pending operation only days away.

## Keys for Taking Control:

✓ Update your health history.
✓ Bring a support person to listen and write responses down.
✓ Discuss surgical expectations and issues following the operation.
✓ Expect a brief physical exam.

\*   \*   \*   \*   \*

THE ACTIVITY FOR TODAY:

*WRITE DOWN TWO FINAL QUESTIONS FOR THE SURGEON TO ANSWER.*

\*   \*   \*   \*   \*

# LINDA'S STORY

*"In an emergency, the most important thing is to have a primary-care physician who knows you and whom you trust. My doctor's quick response and judgement saved my sight."*

**ON** *a beautiful day in September, I sat in a college workshop, enjoying the day and relaxed from an actual vacation in a cabin with no phone, nearly ready to get back to teaching four classes of writing. I have always loved the feel of fall, the sound, the anticipation of students.*

*I had just had an article accepted, had been nominated to the Delegate Assembly of the Modern Language Association, and had finished as Program Chair for the Midwest Regional Conference on English in the Two-Year College. Locally, five of us were in the initial stages of the first freelance writer's conference in Lansing. I was the new president of the Historical Society. When I could, I talked floor-plan designs with my husband, Bob, for his company and sketched designs for his clients, a great satisfaction of a life-long avocation.*

*At the workshop, I slid into a seat beside a friend who taught nursing. At the break, she said, "How are things* going?" It was a routine question. I said, "If I could see the board, everything would be fine," and assured her that I didn't forget my glasses because I had never worn glasses.

She said, "Tell me what you are seeing."

I told her that there seemed to be something in the way of my sight, something fuzzy that I had to look around, like a shadowy thumb in the way.

She said, "When did this start?" I told her that I had noticed it two days earlier, maybe three.

"Have you had any other changes in your eyes recently?" she said. "Spots? Light flashes?"

As a matter of fact, I had. Five days earlier, while driving back from a visit home to divide my grandmother's dishes with six cousins, I had been bothered by diminished sight—and some flashes of light along with black spots.

But for me, these changes signaled the onset of a migraine, migraines so severe that I lost my sight and vomited. I had been working with my doctor for years trying to determine if the migraines were related to stress, food, thyroid deficiency, or early menopause. They had started when I was twelve years old and had occurred occasionally since then. Recently, they were much more frequent, more severe, and of longer duration. I carried medication with me at all times.

She said, "Have you told your doctor?"

I told her that I had spent the morning getting lab tests and a chest X-ray for my annual physical. If my eyes still bothered me, I'd mention it Friday at my follow-up appointment.

She said very carefully, "You will go call your doctor right now and tell him that he wants to see you today."

I calculated all that had to be done at home before I

*sank into classes again. "Can't it wait until Friday?" I said.*

*"Not if you want to see by then."*

*My doctor's response was immediate. "Come in as soon as you can find Bob. Do not drive. We'll wait for you."*

*I didn't have a clue what was happening. I knew nothing about the eyes. At an eye check-up a year earlier, the doctor had assured me that it wasn't quite time for bifocals. Those were the only words I knew. (No, my mother had had a lens transplant, I think, and she suffered from iritis.)*

*Upon exam, my physician explained briefly that my retina in one eye was detaching, and that it would mean surgery. This doctor had been our health mentor for many years. He referred me to an ophthalmologist that he thought was the best. I trusted his judgement completely.*

*The ophthalmologist was very gentle and very concerned. He didn't like what he saw. Because he was leaving on vacation, he referred me to a team of eye surgeons near Detroit, one of the four top teams in the country. He said he would call ahead; we were to go immediately.*

*I began to accept the idea of surgery. Classes wouldn't start for another nine days; this timing wasn't too bad.*

*"Well," I said, "I guess I'd better go pack my toothbrush."*

*"No," he said, "you are not going home. You are leaving now from the office. Your husband will drive very carefully and you will cover your head in the car."*

*We lived three miles away. Finally the seriousness of the situation sank in.*

*"This is not good," I said.*

*"No," he said, "this is not good."*

*"Tell me what I'm in for."*

*He had been waiting. "Your retina is too far detached for laser surgery. You will need invasive surgery, a scleral buckle." He explained the procedure. "If you do not have the surgery right now, we will not be able to save your sight. If all goes well, you will wear glasses and be back at work in about three months. There may be follow-up surgeries needed."*

*Riding to Detroit, I kept my head perfectly still. The blanket over my head protected my eyes from the sunlight.*

*For the next several hours, my whole system was on hold. My worst nightmare had always been that something would happen to my eyes, and now that it was coming true, I simply became a robot and did what I was told to do. Emotionally, I removed myself from what was happening to me. I was in shock.*

*At the hospital, I moved from desk to desk, and office to office in a stupor. I was examined by various doctors at the retinal clinic and again after admission to the hospital. Everyone was terribly careful and they cautioned me not to move my head for any reason.*

*I talked to the surgeon, who explained the procedure again and the uncertainty of the result, then I told the anesthesiologist about my "over-reactions" to certain drugs. I wanted the surgery soon.*

*The surgery was postponed until early the next morning. I was told to sleep on my side, "opposite" the tear in my retina, without moving. The nurse would check me every thirty minutes.*

*In the morning, surgery was postponed again, until noon. I had had no time to prepare for this surgery, and*

*I couldn't prepare for the aftermath until we knew how the surgery went. My eyes were dilated so I couldn't see even with the "good" eye. I was disoriented from the lack of sight, from the exams, and from anticipating the surgery. I knew no one. I developed the beginnings of a migraine, and they couldn't give me anything.*

*But I believed that these kind doctors would do what they could, and Bob was back early in the morning. (He had gone home late at night to make phone calls.) I needed Bob for emotional support, even though there was nothing he could say for reassurance. We simply waited together for the surgery. I tried not to think.*

*I was holding up, as they say, until I went into pre-op and Bob was gone. And then fear and the pre-operative medication kicked in. I began to shake, and shake, and shake. I couldn't control it. I began to cry. A nurse came over, patted my arm, and hollered across the room, "Jan, we need you over here. Case of nerves." Announcing it to the whole room eased some of the fear.*

*The surgery went well, they said. Bob was with me again, and one of my sons had driven to Detroit to be there. When they removed the bandages the next day and held up two fingers, I could see them. I was amused by their primitive test, but we all breathed a little easier.*

*But before I was released they did some follow-up surgery, insertion of a gas bubble, and I couldn't move my head again for a few days. They also explained more fully that the surgery does not reattach the torn retina, but assists it in reattaching itself by changing the shape of my eyeball. The gas bubble would help push the retina back into place from the inside. They would not know what degree of sight I would have for three months. The surgery was "successful," but now it was cross-your-fingers time.*

*I wouldn't be able to read for at least three months. (I was always reading.) I wouldn't be able to teach. (Teaching was my life.) How would this term's students do? I was exhausted from the tension and the anesthetic. I couldn't sleep because I couldn't find any place to put my head that didn't hurt. I couldn't walk without assistance because of the surgical change in my eye, which caused distortion in position and depth perception; any fall could detach the retina again. I was not to bend over. I was not to cough. I was not to lift anything heavier than my coffee cup. For several weeks I was not to do anything at all.*

*I have never felt so helpless, or so useless. I didn't know if it would get better.*

*What if this was it? What if I stumbled through these three months and didn't recover vision? What if the other retina detached? (Not unlikely when it's caused by a genetic predisposition. Other causes had been ruled out: I had not had a blow to the head; I had no family history of retinal detachments; I was not diabetic; I was not extremely near-sighted, in fact, had not even worn glasses before.)*

*Could I teach? Teach writing? What would I do if I didn't teach? How would I ever do design work again? Everything I did depended on my eyes.*

*While I questioned my life, life went on around me.*

*Family and friends came to visit. One friend read to me. Another friend brought me a gardenia, the "smelliest" flower he could buy, because he knew I couldn't see. A colleague signed me up for Books for the Blind from the Library of Congress, a program administered by the State Library, so I could listen to books on tape. I listened to music. I rested.*

*Gradually, I rested enough to feel a little better. I found I could make phone calls, even though I couldn't see* the keys, because all phone keypads are identical. *(Bob would list clients' numbers for me in very large print.)* I realized that, through much experience, I could do floor plans in my head, so I "worked" on a house Bob was restoring after he read me the measurements.

Eventually, my distorted sight became familiar enough to walk outside, carefully. Near the end of the three months, I interviewed several people for an article, by phone. I drafted the article on the computer without being able to read it, but others helped.

And I remembered a student of mine who at 60 had lost his sight entirely from the flu. He was an automotive designer, a pilot and an artist. After two years of physical and emotional blackness, he came into my freelance writing class to learn to write what was in his mind.

I could not fathom what I would do if I didn't regain my sight, but so far I had vision in one eye. At the same time, I knew that there wasn't anything I could do about this situation. What had happened had simply happened, and the result would be whatever it would be, and later, after I had more information, I would make any changes that had to be made.

I was lucky. After three months my retina had reattached itself and healed sufficiently so that I could be fitted for glasses. It took two more weeks for my eyes to adjust to what I saw with the glasses, a small jolt that no one had mentioned, but most of the distortion was corrected and I was allowed to see print again.

Six years later, my retina detached again. This time I knew the signs. I took a careful shower and did some careful ironing. I called the ophthalmologist and packed my toothbrush, knowing that I wouldn't be coming home right away.

*The old scar was in the way, and the surgery took almost seven hours, most of the night. This time, they knew more and controlled the anesthetic somewhat better. They had me do simple breathing exercises to ward off pneumonia.*

*Unfortunately, after two weeks, the new scar tissue went crazy, forming keloids and threatening to pull the retina away again. For six weeks, the surgeons watched my eye, hoping to let it heal as much as possible from the surgery before the scar tissue caused another detachment. I could see less and less all the time.*

*Eight weeks after the previous surgery, the doctor successfully peeled the scar tissue from my retina. Miraculously, I could see the fingers again. This was followed by three minor surgeries: another gas bubble and then two laser surgeries.*

*It all worked, again. After three months, I was back at work, waiting for adjusted glasses. The distortion is greater this time, but I still have sight in both eyes.*

*I have learned it's important to listen to your body. Unusual changes can signal a serious problem.*

*And in an emergency, the most important thing is to have a primary-care doctor, a family doctor, who already knows you and whom you trust. My doctor's quick response and judgement saved my sight.*

*One day, someone said, "Don't you just hate wearing glasses?"*

*"No," I said, "not at all."*

# TALK WITH THE ANESTHESIOLOGIST

*T*here are many types of anesthesia used with surgeries. If you are receiving a general anesthesia, nothing is more important than discussing this procedure with the specialist who will handle your *levels of consciousness* during the operation. You can prepare for this visit ahead of time. This mutual exchange between you and the anesthesiologist or nurse anesthetist is essential for a *safer* surgery.

Ideally, this discussion takes place several days before the procedure or is combined with the pre-operative visit. Some specialists call their clients the day before surgery, but this exchange can be hampered if pre-operative instructions are being carried out at the same time. If possible, an earlier discussion of anesthesia is more helpful.

Regrettably, you do not have control over when the anesthesia for your surgery will be discussed. In reality, this conversation might take place just hours before your operation or in the holding area before being wheeled into surgery. The exchange of information is necessary *before* your pre-operative medication (sedation).

You can always call the department of anesthesiology at the facility where you are having surgery to get questions answered ahead of time. This is helpful, particularly when you will not talk with the anesthesiologist or nurse anesthetist until the day of the procedure.

### *Give Documentation*

Give pertinent health information in writing to the anesthesiologist or nurse anesthetist; have questions and concerns written down. Here are ideas on what information to offer:

*Familiar name*: Give the name you go by that you best respond to.

*Drug history*: If you did well with a certain anesthesia, mention the name. Indicate any *bad reaction* to an anesthesia; give the name of the drug. List prescription or over-the-counter drugs that you are *allergic* or sensitive to. Clarify the medications you are taking. Discuss your tolerance level with drugs. Do you take on-going medications or do you rarely take drugs? Request the *smallest amount* of anesthesia to do the job; this will reduce side effects. Tell the specialist if you and your surgeon have agreed upon the PCA (Patient Controlled Analgesia) device.

*Health history*: List your heart, lung, or other diseases to avoid problems during surgery. If you are being treated for an infection, give that information.

*Other information*: Note if you have given autologous blood donations.

### *Seek Information*

To relieve concerns, ask questions or discuss issues with the anesthesiologist or nurse anesthetist:

1. Ask what types of anesthesia are used with your surgery; which one or what blend of drugs will be used and why? What effects might you expect following the operation?

2. Inquire about the work history of the specialist. How long has the specialist been in the area of anesthesiology within this facility? Other hospitals, other surgical clinics? What are the credentials?

3. Express fears and get questions answered.

This mutual exchange of information is vital to your safety during and following the procedure. Seek resolution of your concerns so that you can go into surgery with some level of calmness.

## *Keys for Taking Control:*

✓ Call the department of anesthesiology to get questions answered if your exchange with the specialist isn't until the day of surgery.

✓ Give key documentation and information prior to sedation.

✓ Ask for the credentials and background information of the specialist.

✓ Resolve remaining concerns.

\*   \*   \*   \*   \*

THE ACTIVITY FOR TODAY:

*LIST ONE IMPORTANT PIECE OF YOUR MEDICAL HISTORY THAT THE ANESTHESIOLOGIST NEEDS TO KNOW.*

\*   \*   \*   \*   \*

# Chapter 14

# PACK, PREP, THEN EASE UP

$S$ome people are hospitalized the evening before surgery and the hospital staff guides them through the preparation for the operation. But this is rare today. More than likely, you will prepare yourself and will check in at the facility on the day of the surgery.

Consider three tasks that need to be completed:

- ► The packing of necessary items.
- ► Completion of surgical preparation.
- ► Relaxation and rest.

For same-day (out-patient) surgery, packing is quick and easy. You simply take along a bag for the clothes you wear to the hospital or surgical clinic. Stable shoes and casual, loose fitting clothes are important. With arm or leg surgeries, large sleeves or large leg openings help to accommodate some hand/foot dressings or casts. If you are having abdominal surgery, you want a pair of pants with an adjustable drawstring for the waistband. For women, a bra

for support following a breast biopsy is sometimes necessary.

### *Pack Ahead of Time*

With a major surgery, packing can occur over several
days.  You can leave a small suitcase open and put items
in the suitcase as you think of them.

A list of basic articles should include a robe, slippers,
soap, toothpaste, toothbrush, and comb.  You want a bath-
robe that wraps around you with *large* open sleeves to
accommodate the IV equipment.   Your slippers need a
*tread* to prevent falls; slip-ons are easier to get into following many operations.

With some surgeries, men and women might take
pajamas with a drawstring waistband and large sleeves or
women can take a short nightgown.  For chest or upper arm
surgery, a button-down top with large sleeves can work;
avoid a pullover.  Hospital gowns can be provided but they
lack dignity and there is a cost.

You may bring other items, such as shaving supplies,
toiletries, basic cosmetics, socks, and your own pillow and
pillowcase.   Women with pierced ears might pack one
small, inexpensive pair of earrings.  With permission from
your surgeon, you may take your own prescription drugs or
vitamins and minerals.   Resist bringing in stationery to
write letters or large books to read because the hospital stay
will be brief.

### *Leave Valuables at Home*

Your support person can bring other items as you
need them, but avoid expensive ones, valuables, and money.

An expensive CD player, boom box, or jewelry for example, are best left at home. You might decide to leave your contact lenses at home and only take your glasses. Take an *inexpensive* watch, travel clock, radio, CD or audio-cassette player with headphones.

Include paperwork or other items in your packing, such as your insurance card(s), advanced directives, or blood donation numbers if they were not given to the nurse during the pre-operative visit. If you have written health information to offer or written questions for the admitting nurse or anesthesiologist, take that too. Set the paperwork and suitcase by your door.

### Pre-op Instructions

Preparations for the surgery are next and they vary according to your type of surgery and the time of your scheduled operation. You will be asked to stop all food and liquids at a given time and to stop smoking if you have not done so. For some surgeries, a Fleets enema, shaving, a shower with anti-bacterial soap (to reduce risk of infection), or other procedures might be ordered. With some surgeries, women are asked to use a betadine (povidine) or other prescribed douche.

### Rest and Relaxation

With packing and surgical preparations done, it's time to relax. This might be hard because of your feeling nervous or anxious, which is common before surgery. You might over-react to people around you because of this tension. Try to *avoid* family conflicts because you want to experience some calmness.

It's time to ease up; it's time to let go. Try to take one or two hours to unwind before you go to bed. Mental diversion helps. You might immerse yourself in a book, watch a light TV program, or talk with your support person. You might use music, guided imagery, or a relaxation tape. If possible, you want to drift into quality sleep.

In bed, take control of your thought pattern if your mind is racing. Repeat reaffirming statements, such as "I'll be okay, no matter what," your favorite prayer, calming words, or positive phrases over and over. Imagine your favorite vacation spot and re-visit the experience. You might try *square* breathing: inhale for a count of six seconds, hold the breath for six seconds, blow out the breath for six seconds, then breathe normal for six seconds. Each time you exhale, feel the body relax more.

Don't panic if you can't drift into sleep; you might be trying too hard. Don't worry if you can't stay asleep. It's okay. Remember, rest and relaxation are your goals.

Be gentle with yourself the night before the operation. Your only task in the morning will be to go into surgery with a positive frame of mind and a rested body.

## Keys for Taking Control:

✓ Pack a limited number of items for the hospital. Leave valuables at home.
✓ Include your paperwork with the packing.
✓ Complete surgical preparations conscientiously.
✓ Use techniques for rest and relaxation.

\* \* \* \* \*

THE ACTIVITY FOR TODAY:

*LIST ONE TECHNIQUE THAT YOU WILL USE FOR DIVERSION THE NIGHT BEFORE SURGERY.*

\* \* \* \* \*

# BE READY FOR ADMITTING & PRE-OP

*Y*ou are ready to go to the hospital and your support person is with you. You've completed the surgical preparations and have ceased all fluids and food at the designated time. If you feel anxious, that's all right because most people sense nervousness on the day of surgery.

You've packed key information for the admitting nurse and the anesthesiologist or nurse anesthetist, if this discussion hasn't occurred yet. Consider giving your support person copies of pertinent information, too. This support person can keep the insurance card(s), driver's license, and other items safe for you.

Generally, you need to be at the clinic or hospital, in the admitting area, two or more hours before the scheduled surgery. When you arrive for an in-patient procedure, you might be assigned a bed in a room. But for same-day surgeries, you could be assigned a cart, recliner chair, or a bed in a large room with curtains pulled between patients.

### Review Timing

If you wish, ask to review the sequence of the day with the approximate timing. This information is more helpful to your family members or the support person.

As the nurse reviews your chart, confirm your drug allergies or other vital facts. Your laboratory and other test results should be on the chart, too; you can ask for the results of the tests at this time if you are interested.

If you brought in paperwork, give this to the nurse. Review and resolve any questions or concerns.

### Consent Form

The admitting nurse will review the consent form with you if it hasn't been signed. This form, which differs in every hospital, is called an *informed consent* since your surgeon has already explained the surgical procedure, why it is necessary, how it will be done, and the possible risks.

Read the consent form carefully. This document usually includes your request for the named surgeon (and associates) to perform a specific operation. It often implies your understanding of the surgery, its risks, and possible complications. The consent form might include permission for additional or different procedures to be performed, if necessary, and your understanding of the need for anesthesia and its risks. It could also address a request for videotaping the surgery, removal and disposal of organs and tissue, or other key issues important to specific facilities.

If your operation is written in medical terms, have the nurse print it out in *lay language* above the medical words and explain the procedure. Don't sign the form if the surgery differs from what you and your surgeon have agreed upon. Be assertive if there are problems and request to speak to your surgeon, even if it means holding up the pre-operative medication, other preparations, or the surgery itself.

You may be asked to sign a permission slip for blood or blood products to be used if necessary. For some surgeries, the chance of needing blood is slight. Signing this form is policy in most facilities; in some healthcare settings, it's required for all procedures; exceptions are rare.

### Pre-op Area

In the pre-op area, you'll change into a hospital gown and be given a cap to wear (particularly for major surgeries). An ID bracelet will be placed on your wrist with your name, room number (if known for in-patients), and your surgeon's name.

If you haven't talked to your anesthesiologist or nurse anesthetist by now, ask about this. To a degree, success with your surgery depends upon this exchange of information. It can't be rushed. You want time to have your questions answered and to feel comfortable with this person. This sharing needs to occur *prior* to any pre-operative medication.

The nurse will check your pulse, blood pressure, and temperature, then begin preparations that have been ordered by your surgeon. With some surgeries, you might be shaved in the operative area or have a urinary catheter, called a Foley catheter, inserted. With more serious surgeries, other tubes, such as the naso-gastric (NG) tube are inserted and other procedures are done or completed in the operating room under anesthesia.

You might be helped into special elastic stockings to prevent blood clots. These support stockings also aid circulation. With an arm/leg or other surgeries, you might be given a special marker to mark a YES or NO on the appropriate limb or area to prevent mistakes. Every surgery requires a different preparation. You'll be guided by the nurse and the surgical staff.

An intravenous (IV) line will be started. If you have chosen the PCA (Patient Controlled Analgesia) method of pain control, remind the nurse and anesthesiologist or nurse anesthetist, because it requires different equipment. Most anesthesiologists have a preferred arm in which to start the IV line, but if you are given a choice, choose the non-dominant arm. Take long, deep breaths while it's inserted to limit discomfort.

The IV line allows you to receive continuous fluids before, during, and following your surgery; it prevents you from becoming dehydrated. The IV solution often contains glucose and electrolytes such as sodium, potassium, and other essential ingredients. It also allows the easy administration of a general anesthesia, antibiotics, other drugs, or blood, if necessary.

With many surgeries, you will remove dentures, partial plates, hearing aids, jewelry, hair accessories, glasses or contact lenses, and similar items. You can give these to your support person. Depending upon the type of surgery and the facility, you may be allowed to keep some items for minor procedures. Most hospitals do not permit nail polish to be worn, since the color of the nails is monitored during some surgeries as one indicator of circulatory problems.

### *Pre-operative Drugs*

Pre-operative medications are important and often include a sedative drug, a narcotic drug, and/or an anticholinergic drug. These drugs relax you, soothe anxiety, prevent secretions from accumulating in your windpipe, ease the surgery, and prevent surgical complications in some cases. They also help the anesthesia work better. Because these drugs make you drowsy and mentally affect you, the signing of the consent form and the anesthesiologist's visit need to *precede* this medication.

### *Holding Area*

You might go into a holding area from 30 minutes to one hour before the actual surgery, or you might stay in your room or cubicle. Once you are separated from your support person, you can always speak to a nurse or surgical team member for reassurance. If you are cold or shaking from nervousness, ask for blankets. Many hospitals keep the blankets warmed; this warmth calms you immediately. Last minute details and final procedures take place this last hour.

The admitting experience affects surgical success. This is a time for you to release control, accept guidance, and move through the surgical process. Make sure your concerns are resolved and you feel comfortable going in for surgery.

## Keys for Taking Control:

✓ Read your consent form carefully. Sign it when you are comfortable with the wording.

✓ Hold back the pre-operative medication if your consent form isn't signed or you haven't talked with your anesthesiologist.

✓ Keep your support person with you as long as possible.

✓ Release control and accept guidance from the surgical team.

\* \* \* \* \*

THE ACTIVITY FOR TODAY:

*CHOOSE THE SUPPORT PERSON WHO WILL BE WITH YOU FOR THE DAY OF SURGERY TO OVERSEE YOUR NEEDS.*

\* \* \* \* \*

# PULL ON YOUR COPING SKILLS

*Y*ou might feel calm on the day of surgery. Perhaps admitting goes well, the surgical staff helps you, your support system is reassuring, the pre-operative medication brings a relaxed mood, and surgery is on time. Everything moves along smoothly.

But in reality, this day can bring tensions and sensitive feelings. If repeated concerns bombard you, it's difficult to manage them. Each new problem can overwhelm you and drain away needed energy. Resolve these issues quickly.

Changes happen. For example, your time of surgery can be altered immensely. Surgeries are cancelled. Emergency surgeries are added. Surgeries turn out to be more complicated than planned; surgeries go more smoothly than anticipated. Surgeries are moved up and surgeries are moved back. Schedules change constantly in this department.

### Stay Flexible

Keep your expectations realistic on the day of surgery. Expect changes to occur because that is what happens. It is healthier for you to *adapt* to the shifts than feel increasingly frustrated when you are already uneasy.

Try to stay flexible because this helps you to manage what is happening. Do your best and pull on your support system. Your ability to adapt influences the nervousness you feel. Ride the waves of change.

### Emotions

Last minute emotions can bombard you. You might flood with loneliness. Although nurses and other surgical team members scurry around, you may feel detached from this whirlwind of activity.

Feelings might intensify. Fears and doubts can creep in. You might regret the decision to have surgery, feel an urgency to have the operation over with NOW, shake from nervousness, or flood with tears. These responses are more likely if you are alone or have not received your pre-operative medication.

Manage these feelings by talking with a nurse or another surgical team member. If you are cold or have the shakes, request extra blankets. The warmth may calm you.

### Strategies

Other strategies can soothe the situation. They will divert your mind, help you to focus, and relieve some of the emotional intensity. Try blanking your mind, a technique in which you visualize the back of your forehead as a blackboard. See the word RELAX written in white chalk on the board, then focus on that word until your body relaxes. Keep re-focusing if your mind is racing.

You might pass the time with a game of countdown by repeating the statement, "In four more hours, this surgery will be over." Or you could comfort yourself by repeating an affirmation, such as "This too shall pass," or reciting a calming prayer over and over. Using imagery, you could mentally remove yourself from the area by reliving pleasant memories.

To release mental, emotional, and physical strain, try deep breathing. Each breath takes only a few seconds. Count up to six while taking in a deep breath through the nostrils, hold the breath for six seconds, then count down from six while *slowly* blowing out the breath. When you combine breathing and counting, the benefit doubles.

Relaxing your body also eases strain. Starting with your toes, tell your muscles to *release* any tension. Move up your body to other muscle groups (legs, thighs, abdomen, back, chest, hands, arms, shoulders, and face), and command each group to let go of any tightness. As each set of muscles relax, remind yourself, "My body is *heavy* and *warm*." This is a powerful exercise, especially if you are cold, because it can warm you.

### *Support People*

If you stay in the admitting area with your support people until you go to surgery, you can express your needs and get reassurance whenever you choose.

When you are taken to the surgical holding area or taken to surgery, your support people will stay in the surgical lounge for the extent of the operation. While they wait, if they need to leave the room for any reason, they should tell the staff person in the lounge and specify where they will be. Sometimes unforeseen complications or emergencies arise during a surgery and family members or support people need to be consulted immediately.

Staying flexible and managing change are important tasks prior to the operation. Your overall goal is to go into surgery in a state of calmness to boost surgical success.

## *Keys for Taking Control:*

✓ Stay flexible with changes.
✓ Divert your mind through strategies.
✓ Use techniques to release tension.
✓ Have support people stay in the surgical lounge.

\* \* \* \* \*

THE ACTIVITY FOR TODAY:

*CHOOSE ONE POSITIVE STATEMENT TO REPEAT ON THE DAY OF SURGERY.*

\* \* \* \* \*

# BARRY'S STORY

*"I don't believe in accidents.
I believe that experiences
are put before us as an
opportunity to grow."*

**ON** *a stifling Friday afternoon of 90 degrees and high humidity, I returned home from work early, highly frustrated, and well aware of how over-extended I was at the college.  Something would have to change.  It was August 27, 1993.  My wife, Nancy, and I had been pushing to complete tasks before the cook-out on Saturday.  A long list of projects nagged at me as I raced to get started.*

*First, that 6' x 10' pile of brush in the yard had to go. I plowed through the containers in the garage, grabbed the kerosene can, doused the brush pile in three spots, lit the match, and tossed the flame in.*

*The explosion blew me 75 feet across the lawn.  While in the air, I remember analyzing why the blast had happened, since kerosene had always been used to get fires started.  Later it was learned that I had grabbed a gasoline can in haste, not the kerosene container.*

*Landing on my feet and staggering back, I threw myself to the ground and started rolling, with my hair, arms, and legs engulfed in fire.  Nancy rushed me, shaking uncontrollably and in shock, to the emergency room.*

In spite of the shock, my logical mind took over, identifying people to be called and projects to be delegated at work. Letting go of work was impossible.

After a transfer to a burn unit in a second hospital, I was placed in intensive care, and was so fortunate to have a physician from India who had spent the last 15 years as a burn specialist in three different hospitals. He listened patiently to my story and treated me as an individual case, different from his other patients. Our meeting was meant to be.

Over 40% of my body had 2nd and 3rd degree burns. My right arm and both legs had 3rd degree burns; my back, shoulders, and left arm had 2nd and 3rd degree burns. My face was black, and I was bandaged top to bottom. Since the morphine wasn't holding my pain down, the doctor ordered a different pain medication. One night, I stopped breathing several times; my son, Scott, age 26, sat at my bedside to look out for me.

On the second day, my physician ordered whirlpool treatments and warned me that the whirlpool "would be painful." Twice a day, the staff placed me in the pool, the jets of water pounding on my wounds. I still remember the pain.

During this time, I never saw myself as being burned because I created images of a superficial sunburn. This imagery helped me endure what was happening until I improved and started the healing process.

By the sixth day, my frustration was increasing. I couldn't organize my thoughts or focus on anything, which upset me very much. Suspecting the pain medication, I wanted the drug stopped immediately, but the nurses were adamant that the pain medication couldn't be stopped because my pain would be too great.

*"I don't do pain," I insisted. "I don't do pain."
After demanding to talk to the doctor, then discussing the
medication, he agreed on a compromise. The IV shunt with
the pain medication would be left in while oral medication
would be tried. By the 7th night, I was down to one pain
pill.*

*To help my healing, I used visualization. I saw my
back with smooth skin, my arms strong like my pitching
days when I was young, and myself surrounded by an
orange healing light.*

*My daughter, Susie, age 22, became the town crier
down at the college. Because she was a student there, she
strolled the campus daily, going department to department,
and giving updates on my progress to interested co-workers. Everyone was deeply concerned.*

*Surgery was scheduled for the 8th day to debride the
wounds and remove dead tissue. But during the surgery,
my legs wouldn't stop bleeding so the surgery was stopped.
This cancellation was too much for me; I couldn't take the
disappointment and became depressed.*

*Once the tears started to flow, I couldn't stop crying.
While sobbing, I saw myself as a picture frame that
couldn't hold up. The frame just kept collapsing.*

*Nancy was beside herself and asked what she could
do. "Touch me. Rub me," I said.*

*"But I can't because you are completely bandaged,"
she said.*

*"Rub my feet," I said. As she massaged my feet, the
tears flowed even more. The flood of tears would not stop.*

*This event became the turning point in my healing.
The human touch had triggered such an emotional release
that my mood completely changed. It was clear to me that
I wasn't in charge. I said, "God, I'll be your assistant.*

*You tell me what to do. Your will be done."* From that
moment, I let go of trying to completely heal myself; a
soothing sensation embraced me. As I shifted to a positive
frame of mind, this became the neatest day of my life.

While glancing around at the 83 balloons in my room,
I got in touch with the wonderful support that had been
mine since the accident. Every day the hospital staff
brought a cart full of cards and letters to me and the tears
flowed while reading the concerned messages from people
locally and around the world. The cards, short messages,
and long letters touched me deeply.

Prayer chains for me were busy internationally.
Members of the National Orientation Directors and the
National Council for Higher Education called weekly to
check on my progress. My support was overwhelming.

When the nurses came into my room, the 83 balloons
swayed, making me seasick, so Nancy distributed them to
other patients in the burn unit. Many patients had nothing
in their rooms; one of them had no visitors.

Healing came from many sources. With frequent
visualization, I saw my arms and back with blisters, then
imagined the blisters popping and the skin peeling off.
Using audio-cassette tapes of Tibetan monks, I concentrated
on their healing chants, and over time, with practice, I
could remove myself from the bed. The tapes were powerful. Repeatedly, I reassured myself that I was suntanned,
not burned.

For the upcoming skin grafting surgery, my doctor
wanted to measure the extent of the burned areas. But
after cutting off the bandages of my arms and back, he was
amazed at the healing; he commented that he must have
misread the depth of the burns. But the nurses reminded
him of the severe 2nd and 3rd degree burns and told him

*about my visualization. He was receptive to my efforts to assist healing in other ways along with the medical orders. My arms and back would not need any skin grafting which was the good news.*

*But my legs were not healing, so the skin grafting surgery was scheduled for the next week. When I asked him what would have to happen for my leg surgery to be cancelled, he explained that "skin buds" would have to be present within the leg wounds. Following my request to have the skin buds drawn out on paper so visualization could be used, he drew small clusters of dots on paper. My work was cut out for me, because there were only seven days to improve the healing of my legs. I chose my images.*

*This time I imagined the leg wounds as deep valleys, then visualized them slowly filling in until they were level. Then I saw skin buds popping out and the skin covering over the areas. Although one area wouldn't fill in, with constant re-focusing, it did. Taking the visualization further, I saw the physician coming in, cutting off the bandages and saying, "It's healed. It's healed."*

*Physical therapists worked with me twice each day, but I wanted to go to the physical therapy department to do some real healing. They agreed to let me try. I used a wheelchair the first day, a walker the second day, and a cane the third day to get to the department and pushed myself on the stationary bike and other equipment. Everyone was astonished at my rapid progress.*

*The day before surgery, my specialist came in for the final examination prior to surgery. I commented, "I have something to show you." He carefully cut off the bandages, studied my legs for a long time, then said, "It's healed. It's healed. I cannot believe this. How did you do this?" He wanted a copy of my Tibetan tape.*

*"Let's not be too optimistic," he said. "Put him in the tub and scrub him down." The nurses eased me into the tub but were afraid to apply pressure and only gently rubbed my legs. I urged them to scrub harder. The doctor examined the legs again and was in awe. He said, "You have a good Doctor on your team who has more power than me. Whatever you are doing, keep doing it. When do you want to go home?"*

*The nurses took over and quickly ushered the doctor out of the room. The "no graft dance" was about to begin and he would not be allowed to see it. The three nurses danced wildly; laughter echoed throughout the room. Gentle hugs were exchanged. The dance celebrated the miracle—no skin grafting surgery would be done.*

*I was going home. The nurses convinced Nancy of my hospital discharge because she would not believe me because my progress was four to six weeks ahead of schedule. Nancy would bring clothes, but the nurses remembered the bulky pair of Mickey Mouse boxer shorts that my minister and bishop had given me; they removed the shorts from the hospital closet. This was the day to launch Mickey Mouse.*

*Two weeks later, my elastic custom body suit that extended from the ankles to my neck, was fitted. When they told me that I would wear the suit for 18 months, I defied that too. My "superman" suit arrived in October and I got rid of it in March, against all odds.*

*My physician had told me that I could never grow hair nor have sweat glands on my arms and legs again. But by March, the hair was growing which also baffled him. When I showed him, he just said, "I understand nothing and I am glad to learn from you."*

*Although the doctor recommended not to return to work until after the holidays, I started back at the college part-time on October 11 in a new position, having left counseling. On December 1, I resumed full-time work, firmly setting limits and eliminating many committees.*

*My exhaustion continued until July. I listened to my body, listened to my gut, and sometimes went home early. My message to students had always been, "Think with your stomach, not your brain, because your stomach never lies." People at work were highly supportive.*

*With this experience, my life has changed forever. Now I choose where to put my energy and have slowed down. My philosophy on winning has changed; I don't have to win anymore, because winning takes care of itself. There is no such thing as a bad day. Nancy and I travel more now, using B & Bs, enjoying each trip immensely. I'm at a higher level of living.*

*I don't believe in accidents. I believe that experiences are put before us as an opportunity to grow. People need to try everything and anything to heal. They need to accept the love and support from others and search out medical people like nurses and physicians who believe and encourage them. One of my nurses was very holistic and believed in the power of visualization; my physician was exposed to a multiple theory of medicine. I believe we were all brought together for a reason.*

*With imagery, I tell people to "visualize what they want it to be because if the brain accepts it, the body will follow." I encourage people with a religious background to "trust it." I am now deeper in my religious commitment and involved in the on-going study of my religion.*

*Since this incident, I've returned to the burn unit to talk to and counsel other burn victims. My life experience can't translate into other people's lives, but I listen hard to where those patients are coming from.*

When someone is injured, it affects the entire family. I worried about Nancy. Patients can't heal if their energy is being drained by worrying about family members. It was crucial to me that Nancy was being looked after and was getting the support she needed.

Throughout my ordeal, I had a strong need to maintain my sense of humor and have always respected the power of humor in the healing process. Nancy and I purchased and donated 12 comedy videos for future adult patients within the burn unit.

Human touch healed me. It was the jet streams of the whirlpool touching me, the nurses scrubbing me, and Nancy massaging my feet. Life is an exciting journey.

# *TAKE CONTROL AFTER SURGERY*

*T*he day of surgery is a lost day. By the time you are admitted, have surgery, go to the recovery room, then to the hospital bed or return home, the day has been a series of blurs. You remember very little. Taking control might seem impossible, but there are ways to influence recovery. To ease the post-operative period of time, you will have educated yourself and made decisions before surgery about your:
- ▸ Pain control.
- ▸ Support person.
- ▸ Physical activity.

Your immediate goals are to begin healing, return body systems to normal function, and prevent complications.

### *Pain Control*
Patient Controlled Analgesia (PCA) helps patients to take control over their pain management at a time of vul-

nerability. If you chose PCA, the anesthesiologist or nurse anesthetist inserts the correct equipment when your intravenous (IV) line is inserted.

With the PCA device, you push a button which sends medication through the IV line for quick pain relief. The PCA control button is worn on your gown or your wrist. The system is part of the IV pump apparatus at your bedside.

This electronic system has many advantages. It cuts down on the waiting time for pain relief, prevents pain shots, and works faster than injections into your muscle. Studies have shown that patients using PCA generally use *less* medication, thus side effects are lessened.

The surgeon prescribes the drugs, then nurses program the PCA device with the type of drug, dosage, and safe interval for you. Safeguards protect you from an overdose and tampering is impossible due to an alarm and security system. You want the *least amount* of drugs to do the job and you are the only person pushing the PCA button.

If you do not use the PCA system, don't be a martyr and hold back from asking for pain medication. Grade your level of pain on a scale from 1 to 10 and ask for relief if needed. Good pain control *helps healing*; feeling some comfort is key to early physical activity and a more rapid recovery.

### State Needs

As soon as possible, state your needs. If you're cold, ask for additional blankets until you are cozy and warm. Sometimes the operating room temperature is as low as 65 degrees, so a patient's temperature can drop as low as 94.5

degrees during surgery and remain low in the recovery room. Some coolness can reduce bleeding problems and decrease the bacterial count to prevent infection. However, excessive coldness lowers the supply of oxygen in the body, decreases blood flow, interferes with the blood clotting process, and lowers the body's defense against germs.

In one recent study, a group of patients having colon surgery received warm intravenous fluids and air-warmed blankets; they had only one-third the usual number of wound infections as other patients. Warmer operating and recovery rooms may be in the future.

Within hours (or days with major surgeries), take an interest in what is happening to you and increase assertiveness. Ask the staff about your blood pressure, temperature readings, or medications. Inquire why certain lab work, tests, or other procedures are being done. Monitor and take responsibility for your own health care; it is not only wise but necessary.

### *Support Person*

Your support person is vital to you for the first 24-48 hours. This advocate becomes a go-between with you and the professional staff to ensure a *safe* beginning to recovery.

Because some hospitals are short-staffed, this gatekeeper *intercedes* for you when you cannot think clearly and express your needs. If you are in the intensive care or cardiac care unit following a serious surgery, your support person's role is limited; the time allowed with you might be only a few minutes per hour.

### *Physical Activity*

To prevent complications, such as blood clots or pneumonia, move, move, move—as prescribed by your surgeon. Because of your residual anesthesia and narcotic drugs, you may feel uncomfortable, nauseated, or light-headed, but at all costs, start moving. Shift, reposition yourself, pull your legs up, wiggle your fingers or toes, or sit up in bed. With *professional help*, dangle your legs at the bedside or walk a few steps while pushing your IV pole. *Inactivity is deadly.*

Returning your body systems to full capacity takes time because the anesthesia and drugs slow you down and alter urinary and bowel functions. Early activity and walking help to re-establish body functions. If you don't have a urinary catheter in, ask for aids to help you urinate the first few times, such as a warm pan of water for your hand or running water. With abdominal surgeries, Vela-mints® or special teas can get gas moving, so you can add more fiber and shift more quickly toward a regular diet. Ask for what you need.

### *Cough and Breathe*

Coughing and breathing exercises will start right after a major surgery. Although it may hurt, these exercises are crucial to prevent respiratory problems, especially pneumonia. When you cough, protect your incision with hands, folded arms, a pillow, or a rolled blanket. You can breathe deeply and blow out the breath, which provides pain relief and when you exhale, you relax—less pain. After some surgeries, a respiratory therapist might assist you with breathing treatments using a special machine.

Your immediate post-operative period influences how soon and how well you mend. Your surgeon's orders include a variety of medications and procedures to cover any problem following surgery. Take control—first through your advocate, then on your own—because you want a good beginning to the recovery process

---

### *Keys for Taking Control:*

✓ Use good pain control.
✓ State your needs clearly.
✓ Let your support person intercede for you.
✓ Start physical movements immediately.

---

\* \* \* \* \*

THE ACTIVITY FOR TODAY:

*CHOOSE TWO WAYS TO START SMALL BODY MOVEMENTS FOLLOWING SURGERY.*

\* \* \* \* \*

# SECURE GOING HOME INSTRUCTIONS

*W*hether you have out-patient (same-day) or in-patient surgery, you could be discharged from the hospital or clinic before you feel ready. Insurance companies have made early releases a common requirement due to soaring healthcare costs.

How you feel will depend upon many factors: your health status before the operation, the type and extent of the surgery, length and depth of anesthesia, amount of pain medication received (along with your tolerance level), and your reaction to the whole event. Some patients feel better than others and are eager to go home; others may feel light-headed, nauseated, exhausted, or in pain. A throat irritation, felt by some people, is caused from the breathing tube that was in the windpipe during a general anesthesia.

Because of the effects of the anesthesia and drugs, your ability to comprehend the instructions may be limited. Have a support person present to think, listen, and work for you.  This advocate can elaborate on the information and may be asked to sign the post-operative directions for you.

### Post-op Instructions

Your surgeon's final visit could be brief, but will include your discharge order and instructions.  If you have written questions to ask your surgeon, take care of them now and have your support person write the responses. Leave nothing to memory.

If you want your hospital test results for your home medical file, have the physician write an order along with the discharge orders.  Getting copies of test results, which you and your insurance company pay for, is a *patient's right* in many states.  Some medical facilities hold back until a release is signed or the surgeon writes an order.

Get all instructions for home recovery in *writing*; and have them explained.  The nursing staff usually delivers this information, but other healthcare professionals, such as a social worker, physical therapist, respiratory therapist, or dietician can be included.

With some major surgeries, the hospital dietician provides instructions on a diet, then schedules a follow-up appointment.  If you are on a general diet when you leave, you might be encouraged to increase dietary fiber (fruits, vegetables, and whole grains) and fluids (especially water) to avoid constipation problems.  Otherwise, stool softeners by prescription or bought over the counter will help you until the effects of the anesthesia and medications wear off and physical activity increases.

The post-operative instructions, which vary with each surgery, guide you in what you can and cannot do.  They cover issues such as comfort measures, pain prescriptions, information about your incision, personal hygiene, diet, and urinary/bowel concerns. The list also includes the start-up of activities and sets limitations (lifting, climbing stairs, and driving). With more serious surgeries, some instructions may be withheld until after the check-up in the surgeon's office during the home recovery period.

### *Questions To Ask*

The following questions address information you need before going home:

*Pain management*:  Will your pain pills be less irritating and work more effectively if taken with food?  Or should they be taken on an empty stomach?

*Incision*:  What should you expect with your incision?  Should there be a discharge?  What type of discharge is normal from an incision?    When should you become concerned?  Is a dressing necessary or should the incision be aired?  Do the sutures, clamps, or dissolvable sutures need follow-up?  If so, when?

*Personal hygiene*:  When can you shower or bathe?  Can the incision get wet?

*Diet*:  Are there restrictions?  Do you need instructions and follow-up from the dietician?

*Urinary/bowel*:  Are there any special directions?

*Activities*:  What are the *limitations* regarding walking or light exercise?  When can you climb stairs, resume lifting, or start driving?  What about home chores?  When can you resume sexual relations?

*Work*:  When can you return to work?  Do you need to start back part-time?

*Check-ups*:   How soon is the first check-up in the surgeon's office?   For a major surgery, it could be weeks
away; with a minor surgery, it could be days away.

Most surgical facilities have forms covering all of
these issues. But if a form isn't used, it's helpful to know
what questions to ask.

### Signs of Problems

You will want to know *signs* of a possible problem,
such as an infection or other complication.  For example,
an infection may bring increased warmth, redness, or pain
in the surgical area, smelly discharge from the incision, and
increasing fever.  Following an abdominal surgery, signals
to check out might be sharp abdominal pain, bloating, or an
inability to urinate or have a bowel movement.   Your
surgeon will define signs to look for depending upon your
specific surgery.

In case of any severe problems, you need telephone
numbers and/or a pager number to reach the surgeon
*around the clock* for a few weeks following a serious
surgery.  If your specialist is not available for the immediate recovery time, get a *back-up* physician's name and
phone numbers.

### Home Services

Sometimes patients need to return home on oxygen or
intravenous feedings, or need special monitoring, equipment, or treatments.  In some hospitals, the coordination of
services is handled by the discharge nurse or social worker;
in other facilities, home healthcare staff or visiting nurses
evaluate the needs, then coordinate necessary services.

Examples of home services might be physical therapy, respiratory therapy, nursing procedures, lifeline connections, hospice, or overseeing needed hospital equipment. Before discharge, the coordination of services *must* be in place. As your strength improves, physical therapy, occupational therapy, treatments, or rehabilitation can be scheduled outside the home.

For patients who must be discharged, yet cannot return home, *transitional* care units are available in some areas for a limited amount of time. In these units, patients can slowly resume self-care activities. Patients who live alone without family or support persons nearby find these arrangements helpful. For all services, check your *insurance coverage*.

### *Assert Yourself*

If you and your support person feel you are not ready to go home or needed services are not in place, you *must* communicate this immediately to your surgeon and hospital staff. In most facilities, patient representatives are available to assist in delaying your discharge.

Although you may want to go home, being discharged can bring a potpourri of emotions blended with fatigue. Make sure you are driven home, without stops, in a comfortable vehicle that is easy to get in and out of. When your support person gets the prescriptions filled, make sure the drug inserts are included.

Bathe yourself in self-nurturing activities when you arrive home. Healing and regaining your strength are the only goals.

***Keys for Taking Control:***

✓ Have a support person with you on the day of discharge.
✓ Obtain all instructions for recovery in writing.
✓ Know symptoms of complications. Post the surgeon's phone numbers.
✓ Check insurance coverage if additional services are needed.

\*   \*   \*   \*   \*

THE ACTIVITY FOR TODAY:

*LIST THREE QUESTIONS YOU WANT ANSWERED ON THE DAY OF DISCHARGE.*

\*   \*   \*   \*   \*

# *D*RAW
# *B*OUNDARIES

*Y*ou are home.  It's wonderful to be home, but you can feel overwhelmed.  Chances are that you are on a pain medication or other drugs that affect your function.  Thus, it helps to have home issues settled ahead of time.

Hopefully, you defined some boundaries pre-operatively as you prepared the family for what needs to be done, or you secured help if you live alone.  Now is the time to implement those bounds.

### *Firm Up Boundaries*
Boundaries are *rigid* or *flexible* and differ according to the type and extent of your surgery.  To people receiving same-day surgery, setting limits may be less important because they may return to normal activities, including their job, within a matter of days or weeks.  If this is the case, still plan on extra time off in case you need it or the surgery ends up more comprehensive than originally proposed.

With major surgery, boundaries are *vital* and firm. People cannot engage in simple activities for weeks nor resume work outside the home for months. In the case of brain, heart, or serious surgeries complicated by cancer and treatments, full recovery may not occur for years.

Get your priorities straight. Healing and returning yourself to the healthiest state you can are the only real priorities following a surgery. Unless you *back off* and take care of yourself, the return to health, function, and productivity can be compromised. This means communicating limits assertively and being clear about your needs. This means making tough choices. There are many options.

### *Limits*

Establish telephone limits, especially if you have little or no help. The answering machine screens all calls the first few days following a minor surgery and two weeks or more after a major surgery. This is a rigid boundary. Returning home in discomfort or feeling unwell due to the medication or residual anesthesia, you are in no mood to receive telemarketing or wrong number calls. In addition, some men and women have no help when they return home. This tool is a must.

Casual acquaintances, more formal friends, or distant relatives need not call the first few weeks after a major surgery. On the other hand, special friends can check on you frequently to give support. Remember that you have the option of calling anyone, anytime you want. Regarding work, beepers and E-mail are not allowed.

Restrict visits. Before a major surgery, communicate that you will not be receiving visitors the first week or more at home. Exceptions can be made, such as telling your most treasured friends to drop by to boost recovery. Their presence can hasten the recovery process. Be selective. When you start visits, limit them to 20-30 minutes. Regaining strength requires energy. Lengthy visits tire you and drain you of energy, even though the visits are well intended. If people want to drop off a gift, plant, or a meal, that is different.

### *Accept Help*

Ask for help. During calls or visits, if people ask if they can do anything for you, say *yes*! Take advantage of this opportunity to be pampered. For some people, accepting help is difficult, but for once, swallow your pride and allow assistance with small tasks. For example you might ask for a meal to be brought in, a few shopping items to be purchased, or a small errand to be run. Perhaps you would like one load of clothes washed or dishes done. A health-care professional friend might review hospital bills, if they arrive. If you had arm surgery, a friend could write letters; if you had eye surgery, a friend could read to you. Appreciate being pampered and get in touch with how good this feels.

Pull on the three A's regarding chores: AGREE to let go, ACCEPT the job done, and APPRECIATE the effort. Return home fully resolved that you will *relax* household standards and not oversee activities. After a serious surgery, the worst thing you can do is to see tasks that need to be done, feel compelled to start chores, then actually do them. This behavior, driven by compulsions, delays recovery.

### *Body Talk*

Any attempt to overdo is harmful and will set you back. You need rest to allow healing. If you fail to listen to your body's warning signs of irritability or tiredness, exhaustion will *immobilize* you. Listen hard! Remember that if you are living alone or have uncooperative family members, you hire in, ask for help, or let duties slide.

For people returning home with a cancer diagnosis, other issues need to be managed: emotional shifts, decisions on treatments, arrangements at work, and extended help from family members, to name a few. For them, the setting of boundaries is *more* important because decisions need to be made.

Boundary setting hastens recovery. Nurturing and pampering yourself will bring necessary healing.

## *Keys for Taking Control:*

✓ Set appropriate boundaries.
✓ Make nurturing yourself and healing the priorities.
✓ Set limits on calls, visits, and chores; ask for help.
✓ Listen to your body for signs of over-doing.

\* \* \* \* \*

THE ACTIVITY FOR TODAY:

*LIST ONE RIGID BOUNDARY YOU NEED FOLLOWING SURGERY.*

\* \* \* \* \*

_Chapter **20**_

# CREATE A HEALING ENVIRONMENT

*I*n addition to the post-operative instructions, you can hasten recovery by creating a relaxing environment at home that decreases pain and helps recuperation. Research studies have found a damaging link between stress and healing.

### *Stress Impairs Healing*
Psychological tension affects healing by constricting blood vessels. These narrowed blood vessels can impair tissue repair and slow recovery. Stress also depresses the immune system, which decreases the body's ability to fight infections.

In one recent study, participants suffering chronic stress showed lower scores on immune system tests. Immune system cells were less active during stressful times. Healing was delayed. But in the nonstressed group, the people healed nearly 25% faster.

## *Design Your Environment*

You can design your own area for recovery before the operation and assess your stress level while you recuperate. Be creative in how you might increase relaxation during this time. Mentally, you need a positive frame of mind for this helpful environment to work.

In designing your relaxing space, consider colors, lighting, furniture, temperature, and other factors. The blues, earth tones, off whites, and cool greens are most soothing. Full spectrum lighting, which mimics sunshine, a dimmer switch for subtle adjustments, or a sun porch can be helpful.

Consider the furniture, too, because your needs are unique. You might lie on a comfortable sofa, in a recliner chair, on a warm waterbed, or on a recommended firm or soft mattress. The arrangement of the furniture is more important. Use a relaxing focal point: face a window overlooking a natural setting, watch a gas log fireplace fire, concentrate on a soothing picture, or enjoy a bouquet of fresh flowers.

## *Nature*

Focus, then concentrate on nature—it's so powerful that it can actually change your brain waves! It can produce more alpha waves in the brain, important for wakeful relaxation. In one study in Sweden, photographs of nature featuring water hastened hospital-room recovery rates for heart patients. Those patients spent fewer days in the hospital, required lower doses of pain medication, and experienced less anxiety after surgery than patients in rooms with blank walls or abstract paintings.

Ceiling fans are excellent, not only for circulating the air but for imitating a gentle breeze for a more natural setting. Fresh air is healthier. Surround yourself with live plants. In addition to their natural beauty, they cleanse and detoxify the air and increase the oxygen in your surroundings. A golden pothos is one example of a good filtering plant.

Good ventilation and the right room temperature also affect healing in a positive way. Your environment should not be too hot or too cold. Extreme coldness constricts blood vessels, which delays the healing process. Warmth dilates blood vessels to increase your circulation, which assists healing. With some surgeries, a warm heat lamp might be relaxing.

### *Soothing Sounds*

For relaxation, choose natural sounds: waves crashing against rocks, sounds of sea gulls, bubbly brooks, waterfalls, gentle rains, thunderstorms, crickets, birds singing, or whale sounds. Audio-cassette tapes or CDs of these sounds are available in the environmental section of music, department, wellness, and nature stores.

Music holds magical powers in changing mental, emotional, and physical responses. Studies have demonstrated that slow music can relax; fast music can invigorate. Research has shown that music during surgery is helpful to the patient and to the surgical team. Music therapists have found that the right music can ease pain, reduce blood pressure, lower heart rate, and decrease levels of stress hormones, such as cortisol. From classical to country, choose what pleases you.

## *Smells Make Scents*

To relax, try specific aromas that can ease tension, stimulate you, or prompt positive memories. Smells influence moods and emotions because the olfactory area in the brain is close to the emotion-producing area. Certain scents release the body's self-healing processes.

Aromatherapy, built on a 5,000-year-old tradition, is now used to treat stress, anxiety, and insomnia. Scents of vanilla and lavender calm people; peppermint stimulates. Smells of apples and cinnamon or fresh bread help people recall pleasant memories. Lighting candles with a relaxing smell, enjoying a warm, relaxing bath with scents, or having a massage with aromatic oils (well into recovery) might be helpful.

## *Directed Breathing*

Breathing exercises also help recovery. Directed breathing (inhaling deeply, holding the breath momentarily, then blowing out the breath slowly) can profoundly relax the mind and body. These slowing down effects can be measured by taking your pulse before, then after several minutes of breathing exercises.

Following surgery, muscles contract in response to discomfort, thus increasing the pain experienced. Deep breathing releases this tension, thus *lessening* pain. Concentrating on breathing also diverts the focus from the postoperative discomfort.

Today, pain clinics teach breathing exercises; health care providers now prescribe directed breathing for fears, anger, anxiety, and nervousness, as well as for medical problems, such as asthma or panic attacks.

### *Laughter*

For centuries, humor has been used for surgical healing.  Laughter, called internal jogging, pulls in oxygen, relieves tension, increases circulation, stimulates the immune system, and releases brain chemicals (beta-endorphins and catecholamines) that decrease pain.  Watching comedies on television or reading humorous books may assist the healing process.

### *Pets Can Heal*

Research has shown that patients who have a pet at home recover quicker in the hospital, leave the hospital sooner, and recuperate faster at home.  Stroking pets or talking to animals relieves stress and creates a state of relaxation.  The companionship of a dog or the purring of a cat can bring instant positive responses which hasten healing.

In one study involving single women and their pet, blood pressure decreased an average of 20 points, particularly with women in their 70's.  Having a close bond with a pet can help recovery.

You can create a healing environment at home.  With the right frame of mind, positive surroundings, and relaxation, your recovery can be eased and shortened.

## Keys for Taking Control:

✓ Understand the relationship of stress to healing.
✓ Have a positive frame of mind.
✓ Create a healing environment using a variety of methods.
✓ Relax yourself to let the environment work for you.

\* \* \* \* \*

THE ACTIVITY FOR TODAY:

*IDENTIFY ONE IDEA YOU WILL USE TO CREATE YOUR OWN HEALING ENVIRONMENT.*

\* \* \* \* \*

# JUDY'S STORY

*"I realized that I would only die if I did nothing and I had never chosen to do nothing in my life."*

*CANCER is very scary. People don't know what to say; there is no script. I encouraged people to ask questions and discuss my cancer because that helped me to process what was happening to me.*

*In October 1994, while doing a routine breast self-examination in the mirror, I spotted a dimple in my left breast. As I pushed on the area and felt a small, hard lump, shock and disbelief hit me. Two more times I pushed on the lump, not believing what had been found, and I promptly made an appointment with my gynecologist.*

*When both the mammogram and ultrasound confirmed the lump, my physician referred me to a surgeon for a needle aspiration. Since the aspiration of the breast lump was unsuccessful, a breast biopsy was scheduled within two weeks.*

*Time became a whirlwind. There wasn't enough time to feel comfortable with what was happening, yet there was plenty of time for anxiety to set in. Even though time was flying, I wanted to put time on fast forward to get the biopsy over with as soon as possible.*

*Despite the turmoil, I took control of what I could and did fast and furious reading about breast cancer, surgical options, and treatments. The information gave me confidence in making decisions and knowing what to expect. It was comforting to talk to acquaintances who had had the surgery. My next task was to get my home in order.*

*On the day of surgery, deep breathing techniques eased my nervousness and relaxed me. Our family minister led a prayer which was comforting; I never felt alone because I knew that God was with me.*

*Because of my difficulty of coming out of the anesthesia with a former operation, I discussed this thoroughly with the anesthesiologist. She offered to use a different combination of drugs.*

*During the breast biopsy, a growth of less than one inch was removed. Afterwards, the surgeon told my husband, who told me, that the tumor looked like it was cancerous. Emotionally, I didn't react to the news because of denial. The pathology report would be in his office the next day and I would need to be there.*

*That night, my mind played tricks on me. On the one hand, I told myself that the report on the tumor was probably going to be okay. But on the other hand, I knew that my surgeon had thought it looked cancerous and he was an expert; it was confusing.*

*The next day, my surgeon, noticeably uncomfortable, gently told me that the lump had been cancerous. He proceeded to tell me all of the treatment options, but I don't recall hearing them. That day, I lost it. I hadn't had time to prepare myself mentally and emotionally for the surgery, so this particular part of the process was a very sad one. I didn't worry about the sadness, because I felt that the feeling was appropriate.*

*Decisions had to be made regarding treatment plans and my job. As an elementary school teacher, I had to find a quality substitute teacher and make out detailed lesson plans. Luckily, the people at the school were highly supportive.*

*This was a hard time because of the number of decisions that had to be made, the seriousness of the situation, my depression, and the discomforts due to the surgery. Further tests (bone scan, CAT scan, and chest X-ray) were done to see if the cancer was confined to the breast area or had metasticized. All of the tests came back normal. The pathology report on the tumor indicated that more breast tissue needed to be removed, so a second surgery was scheduled to remove additional breast tissue and to get a lymph node sampling at the same time.*

*My surgeon had explained that the tests done on the lymph nodes would determine whether the cancer had spread. If it had, I needed to decide if I wanted to have my breast removed, or, if the nodes were clear, have extra breast tissue excised, followed by radiation and chemotherapy. They found the lymph nodes clear of cancer, and my disease was called a Stage I, which meant that I had an excellent chance of survival and not having the cancer return. I felt relieved and chose to have the radiation and chemotherapy.*

*Following the second surgery, visiting nurses came to my home for several days to change the dressing and suggest comfort measures. They cared how I was functioning as a person and encouraged me to take pain pills regularly to feel better and move easier.*

*My physical therapist had wanted me to do 7-10 repetitions of several arm exercises which were difficult because my arm HURT! Instead of doing none, however,*

*I started doing three repetitions of each; little by little the repetitions increased to ten.*

*Emotional conflicts played havoc in my mind. Fears that the cancer had invaded my body and that I would meet my mortality plagued me. I was not ready to die. I grieved and felt sad.*

*My grieving wasn't because my breast had been cut; the incision was barely noticeable. For that, I was relieved that a scar could save my life. But I grieved because my life would be put on hold for the next year and my plans to complete a degree would be set aside.*

*At a university breast clinic, I received more information about breast cancer from another surgeon, a radiologist, and an oncologist. Each one looked at my test results, then conferred with my husband and me. They proposed a team approach to my treatment plan, which was a very positive experience.*

*However, during this conference, one of the team physicians was unwilling to answer my questions. He would tell me I didn't need to know or didn't need to know now. But statistics, options, and knowing what could likely happen if those options were chosen were critical to me and I wanted things right out on the table. He wanted to wait.*

*I wanted to know if there was any link between my breast cancer and the fertility drug taken before my first pregnancy, because this might be crucial. If there was a link, then my sister and daughter would not be affected and fears could be lessened. If there wasn't a link, their turn for breast cancer could come later.*

*He still continued verbal pats on the head while telling me "you don't need to know that," or "it really doesn't matter where the cancer came from." But I would have preferred him saying, "I don't know, but I'll try to find some information for you," or "I don't know." This period was full of panic because he wouldn't respond, so the team members referred me to another oncologist with an excellent reputation, who was upfront with me and good at explaining tests.*

*Tough times hit me during the radiation and chemotherapy treatments. One difficult day, on the way to the hospital in the car, I asked myself out loud why I had chosen the hard route. The radiation treatments were giving me a burn and a rash and I was fatigued. Why hadn't I just had the breast removed? Then I reminded myself that I had chosen this option, because statistically it was better for me in the long run. I didn't want to go through all of this again.*

*On the days of feeling good, I walked and the rhythm kept me going. While walking, I created a "Lucky" list in my head. I was lucky because I had comfortable walking shoes, my arm was feeling better, the cancer was found early, the tumor was small and the cancer hadn't spread. Statistics were excellent for recovery, my support was overwhelming, our family had insurance to cover the treatments, I had cooperation from work, and the builder had finished our cottage up north.*

*I also made out my "Yucky" list. I should not have had breast cancer, no one in my family had it, it was unfair, I had always taken excellent care of my health, all of my plans were wrecked, and the disease was life-threatening. As I analyzed these statements, I could move some over to the "Lucky" list, such as my excellent health which helped me to recover faster. I realized I would only die if I did nothing, and I had never chosen to do nothing in my life!*

My goal was to stay focused on things I could do. Some things I could do for a short duration, some things could be done with adjustments, and some things had to be postponed until I felt better. Gradually, I began to do little things, like setting the table or picking up the house. This helped me keep my sanity and made me feel productive.

Our family was struggling, which made me feel bad because many adjustments had to be made. Initially, family members were very supportive, but over time relationships became strained. As a salesman who traveled for his job, my husband found it difficult to be home, taxi the kids, do the housework, and take care of me.

Our children, a son, age 15, and a daughter, age 12, couldn't comprehend my needs and sometimes found the inconveniences unfair. Too much communication about my illness turned them off, but too little talking could not bring about an understanding of my needs. If the treatments had taken one month, we would have been fine, but after nine months of treatments our family could not handle the stress gracefully anymore. Eventually our family sought counseling.

I reached out for support. In time, my daughter helped out, asked how I was doing, and gave affection. My sister was wonderful; she supported me with physical help, obtaining literature, and a listening ear.

Looking back, I should have accepted more overall help. People were very encouraging and willing to help me, but I couldn't always focus and sort out what needed to be done. Joining an excellent support group helped me; it was upbeat and inspirational.

Over time, I returned to teaching and worked as much as possible, because the positive interactions with the children and the adults kept my mind occupied. When it *became difficult to work, I took a leave of absence. However, during all of this, I completed my additional degree.*

*For other women with breast cancer, I would encourage them to get expert advice and treatments from professionals they trust. Also, concentrate on the things you CAN do, accept help from others, and rely on your faith to get you through the tough times. Think about the long-term results; discomfort is temporary. It's a L-O-N-G temporary but still a short pay-off in the scheme of life.*

*Cancer changed my life and I've grown from the experience. Now I do more mental sorting and ask myself "Is this REALLY important? Am I doing this activity because I enjoy doing it or because I've always done it?" Most of life's tasks are really mundane, not priorities.*

*Having cancer reminded me how strong I really am. Today, I plan more opportunities for fun. My husband and children have continued to help out more. My "Lucky" list is longer.*

*I'll be a cancer patient for the rest of my life and will be seen by my physician regularly so future problems can be spotted early and treated quickly. I'll be okay. Time alone is a healer.*

# VISUALIZE
# HEALING

*Y*ou can ease your recovery by blending your imaginative powers with your post-surgical instructions. You can create images in your mind that flood your inner being with warmth, energy, healing, and relaxation. Imagery melts body tension, thus dilating your blood vessels, which increases body circulation and speeds healing to the surgical site. This relaxation also stimulates the production of natural "killer cells" called T-cells that prevent or fight infections.

### Create Images
Visualization takes practice, but once learned, can be a powerful skill for altering mental, emotional, spiritual, and physical states. You can learn imagery by trying the following steps:

1.  Put the answering machine on or unplug the phone. Tell people at home that you are not to be disturbed.

2. Seek a quiet environment and get comfortable (use your prescribed pain medication if necessary).
3. Gently close your eyes.
4. Empty out your mind. Visualize the back of your forehead as a blackboard and erase any mental clutter. Or, divert the brain by breathing deeply for a few minutes and concentrating on your chest and abdominal movements.
5. Choose vivid mental images that you associate with positive results for a focal point.

The best images come from your own experiences. For example, imagine the sun shining down on you at your favorite beach or visualize the waves rolling onto shore, then receding. Concentrate on the image of your choice and re-focus on the picture if your mind becomes distracted. Try visualization for 20 minutes, once or twice daily. Many people use this technique frequently during recovery.

### Sensory Experiences

After several days of practicing visual imagery, add sensory experiences. At the beach, you could feel the hot sun penetrating every muscle in your body, hear the sea gulls, feel the gentle breeze brush you, smell the seaside aromas, or taste the salty air, if at an ocean. As you bask in the warm sunshine, note the increased body warmth and relaxation. You have the power to increase your body temperature; this physiological change can be measured.

### Personal Images

You can personalize the imagery, depending upon your specific operation. As you focus on the body organ, tissue, or area where you had surgery, you can vividly see positive results happening to hasten healing. As an example, you could picture your blood vessels becoming larger and blood flow increasing around the surgical area to quicken healing or see armies of white blood cells marching to the surgical sight to prevent infection. If you are in pain, you could see the pain as a knotted rope, then imagine the knot slowly coming undone, bringing relief to your discomfort so healing can take place.

Some people with cancer combine imagery with their radiation and chemotherapy treatments using a three step process. First, they achieve a deep, relaxed state; second, they picture the exact area of the cancer; third, they imagine a specific treatment working. They might picture a bright light zapping the cancerous area or a cancerous tumor shrinking during radiation treatments.

During chemotherapy, they might imagine healthy blood cells gulping up cancer cells in the bloodstream or good cells viciously attacking weaker, cancerous cells, eliminating them. Visualization never replaces prescriptions or medical practices, but it does blend well with medical instructions following surgery. Trying imagery is a personal choice. To work more effectively, it requires a positive attitude and belief system.

### *Combine Techniques*

Imagery becomes more powerful when combined with other techniques, such as deep breathing and coaching statements. While inhaling deeply and seeing a bright, healing light of energy coming into your body, you might say, "Energy in." When exhaling slowly and imagining a cloud of grey tiredness leaving your body, you might say, "Tiredness out."

Every hour during waking hours for the first two weeks after the operation, you might scan your body for discomfort and assign a specific color to any pain. Practicing your breathing exercises, you could inhale, then hold your breath while scanning your body for any discomfort and see the pain in the color you have chosen. While blowing out the breath, you can visualize the color (pain) flowing out of your mouth, rushing down your hands and out your fingers, rushing down your legs and out your toes.

### *Relax to Heal*

Relaxation for healing can come visually in other ways. You could picture warm, thick honey being poured over your head, which warms and relaxes you as it moves slowly down your body increasing your circulation. While using healing visualization, you might repeat affirmations, such as, "I'll be gentle with myself to help healing" or "Each day I am stronger and healthier." These techniques are very powerful.

For some patients, visualization can be awesome when blended with medical care (see Barry's story, page 104). With the muscle relaxation and increased circulation that imagery creates, healing and recovery are enhanced. It takes commitment, persistence, and practice, but the rewards are great for a select group of people.

## *Keys for Taking Control:*

✓ Consider visualization along with medical instructions.

✓ Create images with specific positive outcomes.

✓ Combine sensory experiences with the imagery.

✓ Use visualization with other relaxation techniques to help your recovery.

\* \* \* \* \*

THE ACTIVITY FOR TODAY:

*CHOOSE ONE POSITIVE IMAGE TO FOCUS ON DURING RECOVERY.*

\* \* \* \* \*

# REBUILD YOUR BLOOD

$D$uring some surgeries, patients suffer a blood loss that decreases the number of red blood cells in the blood. These red blood cells contain hemoglobin, an important substance that carries oxygen in the bloodstream. A serious problem can develop if more and more blood is lost and the level of hemoglobin drops.

Iron, an important mineral, combines with protein and copper to make hemoglobin. In addition to energy production, iron is necessary for sustaining body enzymes, regaining your strength following surgery, and maintaining a strong immune system to prevent infections after an operation.

### Iron Deficiency

Some people fall short of adequate iron intake: some vegetarians, dieters, long-distance runners and endurance athletes (especially women), and pregnant and menstruating women. In fact, several studies have concluded that up to 50% of young women do not consume enough iron during their reproductive years. Certain diseases and infections can also create problems within the blood. Internal bleeding, uterine bleeding, autologous blood donations, or occasional bleeding during or following surgery can cause iron, hemoglobin, and red blood cell inadequacies.

Iron deficiency, the most common cause of anemia, brings complaints of fatigue, irritability, poor concentration, shortness of breath with exertion, increased viral infections, headaches, nail changes, or complaints of feeling cold. Stress increases the symptoms of anemia.

Your physician can define your iron needs with laboratory tests such as a Complete Blood Count (CBC), partial blood count, hemoglobin (Hg) or hematocrit (Hct). Occasionally, other tests are needed.

### *Iron Sources*

If your tests indicate an iron problem, ask your surgeon, the staff nurse, a nutritionist, or a dietician for guidance in building your blood back up. Good food sources for iron include: eggs, fish, poultry, liver, lean meats, green leafy vegetables, whole grains, and enriched cereals and breads. Other sources are: dates, raisins, dried prunes, lima beans, blackstrap molasses, pears, rice, wheat bran, almonds, and soybeans.

If the need for iron supplements exists, ferrous sulfate is sometimes tried first because it is absorbed better along with increased Vitamin C. There are several other iron compounds. All iron supplements must be kept out of the reach of children because they are toxic.

Even though iron is absorbed better on an empty stomach, you need to take it with food or after meals if it upsets you. Cramps, diarrhea, or constipation can be side effects. Increasing exercise and water intake can help prevent constipation. Report severe symptoms to your physician.

Take the supplement with one full glass of water or diluted juice. Liquid iron is taken in diluted juice and sipped through a straw to avoid staining teeth. Avoid taking iron supplementation with milk, tea, or coffee. With meals, drinking tea can block iron absorption up to 85% (because of the tannins); drinking coffee can reduce absorption by 39%. Calcium supplements or excessive amounts of zinc and Vitamin E reduce absorption.

Increasing iron to build up your blood takes time. Only a part of dietary iron is absorbed, with iron from animal sources being absorbed more easily than plant sources. You can increase the iron content of a meal about ten-fold by simmering food and sauces in an iron skillet, the longer the better.

There are vitamins and minerals that aid iron uptake, such as Vitamin C (citrus fruits, potatoes) and A (orange vegetables, milk), the B-complex vitamins (fish, sunflower seeds, milk), copper (seafoods, eggs), and manganese (whole grain cereals). Your stomach also needs adequate levels of hydrochloric acid.

### Recheck Blood

Your blood should be rechecked after four to six weeks on iron therapy. If the test indicates a residual problem, more testing or a different iron compound may be prescribed. Following autologous blood donations and major surgeries, iron needs can increase considerably due to the blood loss.

### Excess Iron

Controversy has surrounded the intake of iron today since a Finnish study in 1992 raised fears about high levels of the mineral increasing risks for heart problems. Several follow-up studies, including one from Harvard, have not found that relationship. More than one million Americans with a hereditary disease called hemochromatosis do need to be concerned with excess iron, which if left untreated, can lead to arthritis, cirrhosis of the liver, or heart disorders. Further studies need to be done to settle this controversy.

Building up your blood, if needed, is crucial. Let your surgeon test and guide you in your iron needs so you can gain strength, increase your energy level, heal better, and assist your recovery process.

## Keys for Taking Control:

✓ Have your blood checked following a surgery with blood loss.

✓ Rebuild your blood, if needed.

✓ Understand dietary and other factors that can block iron absorption.

✓ Get your blood rechecked six weeks into iron therapy.

*   *   *   *   *

THE ACTIVITY FOR TODAY:

*CIRCLE THE FOODS YOU EAT REGULARLY THAT ARE GOOD IRON SOURCES.*

*   *   *   *   *

# Chapter 23

# RESUME YOUR LIFE S-L-O-W-L-Y

*I*f you are wise, you will *slow* down after surgery to allow healing, regain your strength, and refill your energy pool. You can bathe yourself in self-nurturing activities and sense how wonderful that feels. After a major surgery, your full energy level may not return for a long time.

Even if everything goes right, having an operation can throw your mind and body into a state of imbalance; it takes time to re-center yourself mentally, emotionally, spiritually, and physically. If cancer or another life-threatening disease is diagnosed, you will need more time to stabilize.

### Be Gentle With Yourself

Step back. Smell the roses. Enjoy being. Rest. Sleep. Rest. Sleep. Recall special memories. Rest your worries. Immerse yourself in deep introspection. Re-examine your philosophy of life. Re-evaluate your prior-

151

ities. Relax: listen to music, read, and commit yourself to brief walks. Touch base with your support network. As your recovery progresses, give yourself a gift—a haircut, facial, manicure, or massage. All of these activities re-balance your life.

### Pace Yourself

Eventually, you need to re-enter the world of reality, but go *slowly* as you re-start home, social, and job activities. Resist any urge to plunge into tasks too early.

Listen to your body. Let your mind and body direct the pace and intensity of your movements. Increased dis-comfort, irritability, snappiness, defensiveness, or tiredness are all signs of over-doing. Back off quickly. Symptoms happen for a reason.

Allow extra time for routine care, such as shaving, showering, taking a bath, or doing hair care, because you will tire more easily and these activities will take longer. Following serious surgeries, you may feel exhausted after completing one simple task.

When starting home activities, think about using the work-rest rhythm. Work a little, then stop and take a rest. During this pause, you might nap, call a friend, stroke your pet, use imagery, or just enjoy the moment. Do whatever feels right for you.

Even though your support system is helping you with recovery, start social commitments cautiously. Your friends may be eager to be with you and you may be bored, but be careful in over-scheduling yourself. At first, space out your activities in the calendar and make them for brief periods of time. Then allow a respite.

### *Prevent Energy Withdrawals*

View your social calendar as a checkbook. You need to deposit enough energy so that you don't get overdrawn. Energy can be deposited into your bank by eating right, snacking on healthy foods, walking, pampering yourself, resting, and getting plenty of sleep.

You can *prevent* withdrawals from your energy bank by managing your stress and modifying relationships. For example, you might surround yourself with positive people who energize you and limit contact with people who siphon off your energy resources.

You can guard your bank assets against stress during the day by relaxing periodically. As you relax, your energy pool *floods* with renewal. Listen to music, write a journal, direct your breathing, read a magazine, or do gentle stretching exercises to enrich your day. By preventing withdrawals of your resources, your banked wealth of energy is protected.

In the first month following surgery, schedule three 30-minute periods in your day to deposit energy. Keep this commitment to guarantee spurts of energy throughout the day. If you overtax yourself and deplete funds, you will know it. Pull back quickly.

### *Social Life*

Ease into social commitments. After several weeks at home, let close friends take you for a ride, bring in a meal, or treat you to lunch. Be gracious and accept help. But for more distant people, set specific times for visits. You can always increase contacts to meet your needs throughout recovery.

### *Extra Time Off of Work*

Job decisions will be made before an elective surgery. With an emergency surgery, recommendations follow the operation itself. Your surgeon will guide you with these arrangements.

If possible, take *more* time off than what is recommended. Sometimes an operation becomes more extensive than planned or you do not recover as fast as you thought. It is much easier to call your employer and ask to come back earlier, than to call work and request more time off. Saving up personal days and banking extra hours can help extend your sick time. Some people take a medical leave, so look into the Family and Medical Leave Act. Consult your employer or the personnel office for information.

After a major surgery, it helps to start work on a part-time basis. After several weeks of part-time work, you might resume a full-time schedule. The greatest mistake is to go back too soon into a full-time position. Resume job responsibilities gradually.

### *Don't Allow Guilt*

Take the time to heal adequately and recover before returning to work. Don't feel guilty. Don't let co-workers, supervisors, managers, or family members make you feel guilty for wanting sufficient time off. Resist comparing yourself to a colleague who might have had the same surgery and returned earlier to the job. You are different; your circumstances are totally different. Two cases cannot be compared.

Job insecurities create anxiety in the workplace. Don't allow changes at work, such as a re-organization, downsizing, or merger, to entice you back to work too early. Do not feel compelled to shorten your time off.

### *No Beeper Allowed*

If you have a home business or are telecommuting with your company, communicate to your clients ahead of time that you will be unavailable for a length of time. Be firm in limiting your work hours. Develop a system for *separating* your work life from your personal life and let the answering machine, voice mail, E-mail, or fax machine work for you. Limit E-mail, beeper, or Internet exchanges. You have earned a break.

It is far better to regain your health fully before resuming work. By returning too soon, you may pay a high price to your health, possibly to your life! A relapse or new complications could cost you greatly and demand double the time off. Do it right the first time.

In resuming home, social, and career life, your economic status will play an important part in your decisions. Create, modify, and simplify your life so you can ease back into life healthier.

### *Keys for Taking Control:*

✓ Bathe yourself in self-nurturing activities.
✓ Listen to your body to pace tasks.
✓ Deposit energy into your energy pool daily.
✓ Resume home, social, and job activities cautiously.

\*   \*   \*   \*   \*

THE ACTIVITY FOR TODAY:

*IN YOUR CALENDAR, WRITE IN THREE 30-MINUTE BREAKS PER DAY FOR THE FIRST MONTH FOLLOWING SURGERY.*

\*   \*   \*   \*   \*

# PAT'S STORY

*"I allowed myself to feel
sad, angry, depressed, or
down for periods of time."*

**PEOPLE** *have always called me a positive person.
I think I inherited it from my parents who taught me to pull
on the positive side of a dilemma. Likewise, I have tried to
instill the importance of a positive attitude in my three
children. I have always told them that it takes a lot more
energy to be negative than to be positive.*

*I limit my pity parties and allow myself only one or
two days to be down, depressed or discouraged. Then I tell
myself to "Get on with it!" There is no strength where
there is no struggle. I believe that staying positive can
change situations. Being negative changes nothing. Life is
too precious of a gift to waste on self-pity or second
guessing.*

*I've never questioned "Why me?" but I have won-
dered why I've been challenged with continual health problems over the past decade. When diagnosed with Lupus in
1986, I felt grateful that I had the skin problems only, not
systemic Lupus. My health challenges continued with three
spinal nerve blocks, two lumbar spine surgeries, then
lithotripsy (a shattering of kidney stones) several times.
Little did I know that more health concerns awaited me.*

*In 1992 at the university where I worked, I was climbing the four flights of stairs to my office to get more exercise while the elevator was getting repaired. After several weeks, I felt that someone had a fist pushing on my chest. This alerted me that something was different so I contacted my cardiologist from the mid-80's. The ECG and chest X-ray were normal; however when the pressure continued he ordered a stress test. I was 48 years old.*

*After five or six minutes on the treadmill, the physician rushed me to a cot to lie down. He checked my pulse and blood pressure and was shocked that I wasn't having chest pain or shortness of breath. Within minutes I was having an echocardiogram that showed heart problems.*

*I told the staff that I had to go home and put my house in order, but they wouldn't listen. I wanted my family there. My husband, Rich, was on the road and temporarily unreachable, but Brent, age 16, took over and tried to reach him. He also called Lynley, age 20, who was away at college, and she came immediately after communicating with her professors. Brad, age 23, came too. My support system arrived just in time for my heart catheterization.*

*The physician explained everything. Unbelievably, four of my coronary arteries were 90, 80, 80 and 60% blocked. He clarified that I couldn't have angioplasty because my coronary arteries were crooked—like limbs of a tree. I would need a quadruple bypass surgery soon.*

*Rich assured me that we would all get through this together. He wanted to talk about a living will, but I wouldn't have that and kept saying, "Nothing is going to happen to me. I'm going to be fine. . .but if something does happen, keep me in a coma for awhile just in case." He told me I had been watching too many talk shows.*

For six days, they had me on continuous morphine because the physicians worried I might have a heart attack at any moment. They placed me in the intensive care unit for three days, then in the cardiac care unit to await surgery. One day I was vigorously filing my nails when a nurse rushed in and insisted that I couldn't do that. The filing of my nails was throwing off the monitoring equipment.

The timing of the bypass surgery couldn't have been worse since I was supposed to be having a breast biopsy done on a firm lump in my right breast. My breast surgeon reassured me that the breast surgery would have to wait since the heart surgery had to be done NOW.

Emotionally, I was fine until the night before surgery, because initially I didn't realize the seriousness of the situation. As ten friends and family members gathered around me, it struck me that they were here to say good-bye. Suddenly, the reality hit that I might not survive the surgery. I flooded with tears; the tears wouldn't stop coming. After everyone left, Rich and I talked; then he continued the reassurance by telephone from home.

The quadruple bypass surgery on February 13, 1992, went well. When I woke up in pain I said to myself, "This is the best pain I have ever felt." I had made it. I had survived. I felt nauseated. Since I couldn't talk with the tube down my windpipe, the nurse had me write on her hand. I wrote N-A-U, and she understood and dipped a sponge on a stick in cold water and placed it in my mouth.

She taught me to breathe deeply from the diaphragm, which soothed the nausea as well as the pain. Deep breathing and frequent coughing were critical techniques following surgery to prevent pneumonia. Despite the pain, I forced myself to do the breathing exercises.

*In five days I was discharged. The first thing I did at home was to get a dustcloth and start dusting a coffee table. By the time I had dusted a 12" x 12" area, I fell back onto the sofa feeling completely exhausted. My body was communicating that I had overdone it. My parents and family members took over with the home responsibilities.*

*Soon after returning home, I designed a walking area within the house and I walked two minutes each day. Within a few days, I was outside walking and in one week, I conned my mother into driving me to the mall. Although I wanted to shop and felt that great, she wouldn't let me because she knew that just climbing upstairs to our second floor exhausted me.*

*My breast lump needed to be biopsied so I never returned to work. Following that surgery, when no office staff would give me the pathology results over the phone, I knew in my gut that it was a cancer. My breast surgeon called me that night, confirmed the findings, then told me that it was a slow growing cancer so I had plenty of time to make the right decision. He reviewed all of the options with me.*

*Until the night before surgery, I had chosen to have a lumpectomy, but then that night, I discovered a second hard lump in the area surrounding the nipple of the same breast. I was upset, agitated, and insisted on talking with the surgeon. On April 17, 1992, I had a modified radical mastectomy. My husband supported my decision. I felt grateful there hadn't been any lymph node involvement.*

*I wore an "ice cap" before and after my chemotherapy treatments to prevent hair loss. The ice cap was a knit cap that came to a peak which had been frozen. Actually, I looked like a "cone head." Ten minutes before my IV chemotherapy treatment, I put on a shower cap like device, then the frozen knit cap. The ice cap was left on for another ten minutes following chemotherapy. Treatments took place every 2-3 weeks depending upon my blood count and lasted for six months. MY HAIR NEVER FELL OUT!*

*The breast cancer finding was much more emotional for me than the heart surgery. I'm not sure why, except I felt that my life was more threatened by cancer than heart disease. I allowed myself to feel sad, angry, depressed, or down for periods of time. My religious faith, my family, friends, and entire support network helped me.*

*I'm back at work now. It's been several years since my quadruple bypass and breast cancer surgeries. Those experiences taught me to take time for myself. Before 1992, I put everyone else first and didn't take the time to nurture myself. Now I read, work in the yard when I can, walk up to three miles a day, and value my time with good friends.*

*Despite my continued health challenges and family crises over the last several years, I persist with a positive philosophy. I feel so lucky to have a supportive husband and three children who have helped me surpass it all with their notes, phone calls, surprises, and caring. When I'm tossed more lemons, I just make more lemonade.*

# EPILOGUE

*W*hat about the future of surgery? Exciting changes march on the horizon—partly driven by demands for cost-cutting alternatives and the need for consumers to take a greater responsibility for their health care.

Several positive health movements include less invasive surgeries, high-tech procedures, medical education changes, mind/body studies, integration of other therapies with medical management, and an increase in consumer involvement. All of these changes improve the healthcare system.

Less invasive procedures have brought "keyhole" and no scalpel surgeries with an increase in laser and ultrasonic techniques. Biological "super glue" has reduced bleeding problems in some surgeries; uterine balloon therapy and other treatments that destroy the lining of the uterus have stopped or limited bleeding problems, eliminating the need for hysterectomies in some cases.

In dentistry, high and low electronic signals cancel out pain and discomfort—replacing traditional anesthetics. The patient, through turning a dial, regulates the pain-reducing power during some dental procedures.

When available, a new device, consisting of 18 sensors connected to a computer, will complement other diagnostic tools, such as the mammogram, ultrasound, physical exam, and needle aspiration when suspected breast problems arise. A technician will place the sensors on a woman's breasts to measure the electrical activity of the breasts, then compare the findings to normal levels. Estimates claim that this device could eliminate about 200,000 benign breast biopsies a year.

Using computers, surgeons can now practice difficult techniques over and over prior to performing a complex surgery. With a computerized simulated body, medical students can study and dissect the body dozens of times to learn about the bones, muscles, and tissues—without making an incision.

Computers can project 3-D images of organs for anatomical learning or send impulses through an instrument when bone, tissue, or blood vessels are touched to help surgeons get the "feel" for an operation. All of these new techniques reduce surgical risks and complications.

Along with technological advances, other changes are taking place. In medical schools, such as the University of Virginia Medical School in Charlottesville, medical students are being taught meditation.

In 50 of the 135 medical schools in America, anatomy and biochemistry courses are being supplemented with acupuncture, nutrition, and massage. Hypnosis and bio-feedback have also gained respect within medicine.

Nutritional and dietary therapies to boost the immune system, strengthen the patient, and speed surgical recovery have accelerated. The integration of additional therapies, such as music, visualization, faith, humor, pet therapy, and healing statements alongside medical instruction have also eased the surgical process.

As the future unfolds, there will be a better understanding of the physiological mechanisms that influence the impressive communication among the nervous, endocrine, and immune systems (psychoneuroimmunology). All of the research in this new area of immunology will help us to understand how our thoughts and emotions impact our health and disease states, and how we can coach healing following a surgery.

Surgeons and medical organizations, such as the American Hospital Association, encourage consumers to become their own health manager—to take a more active role in their health care, especially when surgery is needed. Consumer advocacy agencies educate men and women and push them to take a greater responsibility within the healthcare system.

As millions of babyboomers advocate for their aging parent or family member, they, too, will have to become more educated, more informed, and more assertive when surgery is suggested.

But nothing will replace the importance of patient education, a team approach to health care, and the quest for knowledge so that patients can sense some level of control in their health management. With an operation, this empowerment paves the way for a smoother surgical process.

Having surgery must be a collaborative journey. With 80% of surgeries being "elective" procedures, there is time to become an active participant in this experience. As a team member, armed with the right research and information, your surgery can be safer and more successful.

# GLOSSARY

**Acquired Immunodeficiency Syndrome (AIDS)**: A disease involving a defect in immunity that has a long incubation period, is manifested by infections, and has a poor prognosis.

**Adrenalin**: A chemical released by the adrenal glands which increases the speed and force of the heart beat and dilates the airways to improve breathing.

**Advance directives**: See Living Will and Medical Durable Power of Attorney.

**Anesthesia**: The absence of feeling and normal sensation, especially sensitivity to pain as induced by an anesthetic substance, hypnosis, or from trauma.

**Anesthesiologist**: A physician who specializes in the administration of anesthetics and monitors the patient's condition while under the anesthesia.

**Aneurysm**: A ballooning of an artery due to the pressure of blood flowing through a weakened area.

**Angioplasty**: Surgical repair of blood vessels damaged by disease or injury.

**Antibodies**: Proteins that are manufactured by a type of white blood cell to neutralize a foreign protein in the body.

**Aromatherapy**: Inhaling fragrances to produce a desired chemical reaction in the brain.

**Arthritis**: Any inflammatory condition of the joints, characterized by pain and swelling.

**Autologous blood donation**: A blood unit given by a person for their own surgery.

**Basal cell carcinoma**: A malignant tumor that begins as an enlarging pimple-like area that develops a crater, then forms a crust and bleeds.

**Beta-endorphins**: Opium-like chemicals that act on the central nervous system.

**Biopsy**: A diagnostic test in which tissue or cells are removed for examination under the microscope.

**Bypass**: A surgical operation that provides passage of blood around a diseased or blocked part or organ (i.e. heart).

**Calcium**: A mineral that forms bones and teeth and helps with blood clotting, nerve transmission, and muscle contraction. Sources are milk, yogurt, fish with small bones, and dark green leafy vegetables.

**Carcinoma**: A malignant tumor (cancer) arising from cells in the surface layer or lining membrane of a body organ.

**CAT (computerized axial tomographic) scan**: A diagnostic technique in which the combined use of a computer and X-rays passed through the body at different angles produces clear cross-sectional images ("slices") of the tissue.

**Catecholamines**: Various compounds, such as norepinephrine and dopamine, that are secretions or by-products of the adrenal gland that affect the nervous system.

**Chemistry profile**: A test to check the amounts of various substances in the body which must be cautiously interpreted (regarding a disease) if abnormal levels are found.

**Chemotherapy**: The treatment of infections or malignant diseases by drugs that act on the cause of the disorder.

**Chromium**: A mineral that appears to increase the effectiveness of insulin and is involved in the metabolism of glucose for energy. Sources are whole-wheat bread, brewer's yeast, beef, and liver.

**Cirrhosis**: A degenerative disease in which areas of the liver are covered by fibrous tissue and penetrated by fat.

**Complete Blood Count (CBC)**: A blood test that generally checks on white blood cells, red blood cells, hemoglobin, and/or hematocrit.

**Copper**: A trace mineral found in all body tissues that forms an essential part of several enzymes and assists in the formation of hemoglobin and red blood cells. Sources are whole-grain products, green leafy vegetables, and liver.

**Cortisol**: A hormone secreted by the adrenal gland which is involved in the stress response.

**Counselor**: A person who advises and facilitates the mutual exchange of ideas, opinions, and discussions.

**Diagnosis**: The act or process of deciding the nature of a diseased condition by examination of the symptoms.

**Dietician**: A person who works in the application of nutritional science to people both sick and healthy.

**Durable Power of Attorney**: See Medical Durable Power of Attorney.

**Echocardiogram**: A diagnostic procedure to obtain images of the structure, position, and movements of the heart using ultrasound (inaudible, high-frequency sound waves).

**Elective surgery**: Pertaining to a procedure that is performed by choice but which is not essential.

**Electrocardiogram (EKG or ECG)**: A record of the electrical impulses that immediately precede contraction of the heart muscle.

**Electrolytes**: Substances such as sodium, potassium, magnesium, calcium, phosphate, and chloride that play an important role in regulating body processes.

**Emergency surgery**: An operation that must be done in response to a serious situation that arises suddenly and threatens the life and welfare of a person.

**Endotracheal tube**: A narrow plastic tube passed through the mouth or nose into the trachea (windpipe) by an anesthesiologist.

**Enzyme**: A protein that regulates the rate of a chemical reaction in the body.

**Family and Medical Leave Act**: A 1993 Federal act that requires employers to provide up to a total of 12 work-weeks of unpaid leave during any 12-month period for employees due to the birth or adoption of a child or serious health condition affecting the employee or family members.

**Ferrous Sulfate**: A drug (iron preparation) that is used for the prevention and treatment of iron deficiency.

**Foley catheter**: A slender rubber tube with a balloon tip to be filled with air or a sterile liquid after it has been placed in the bladder to drain urine during surgery.

**Gastro-intestinal (GI)**: Of or pertaining to the organs of the GI tract from mouth to anus.

**Glucose**: The body's chief source of energy for cell metabolism.

**Health Maintenance Organization (HMO)**: A plan for comprehensive health services, prepaid by an individual or by a company for its employees that provides treatment, preventive care, and hospitalization to each participating member in a central health center.

**Heart catheterization**: An invasive technique in which a catheter is inserted into a vein or artery and guided into the heart to check the chambers of the heart, the blood vessels, heart output, the heart valves, and other measurements.

**Hematocrit (Hct)**: A test to measure the percentage of red blood cells by volume in whole blood.

**Hemochromatosis**: A rare disease of iron metabolism, characterized by excess iron deposits throughout the body.

**Hemoglobin (Hg)**: A protein substance in red blood cells that carries oxygen from the lungs to the tissue or a test that measures the amount of hemoglobin in the cells.

**Hepatitis**: Inflammation of the liver, with accompanying liver cell damage or death, caused by a viral infection, certain drugs, chemicals, or poisons.

**Hormones**: A group of chemicals, each of which is released into the bloodstream by a gland or tissue.

**Hydrochloric acid**: A strong acid released by the stomach lining.

**Immune system**: A collection of cells and proteins that work to protect the body from harmful, infectious organisms, and play a role in the control of cancer and rejection problems of organ or tissue transplant.

**Immunotherapy**: Regarding cancer treatments, it refers to the stimulation of the immune system to treat cancer.

**Incision**: A cut made into the tissues of the body by a scalpel (surgical knife).

**Independent Practice Association (IPA)**: A pre-paid health service system in which office-based physicians contract for the care of patients on a pre-negotiated fee-for-service basis.

**Informed consent**: A careful explanation provided before surgery and where the patient is asked to state that he or she understands the procedure and the risks involved, and that he or she consents to it.

**Interferon**: Proteins produced by some cells in response to viral infections or a foreign particle, which also seem to have anti-tumor properties.

**Intravenous (IV)**: Within a vein, as in a slow introduction of a volume of fluids into the bloodstream.

**Lithotripsy**: A procedure that uses shock waves or ultrasonic waves to break up kidney stones for excretion.

**Living Will**: A written statement that informs the physician and family members of the type of medical care desired or to be withheld if he/she becomes terminally ill or permanently unconscious and cannot communicate decisions.

**Lobular carcinoma**: A tumor that often forms a diffuse mass and accounts for a small percentage of breast tumors.

**Lupus**: A chronic disease that causes inflammation of connective tissue, which can affect the skin and/or organs or systems of the body, especially joints and the kidneys.

**Lymph node**: An accumulation of tissue that is the main source of lymphocytes (white blood cells) which serves as a defense mechanism to remove bacteria and toxins.

**Lymphocyte**: Any of a group of white blood cells of crucial importance to the immune system.

**Malignant**: A term used to describe a condition that tends to become progressively worse.

**Mammogram**: An X-ray procedure to detect breast cancer at an early stage.

**Manganese**: A trace mineral that plays a role in activating numerous enzymes. Sources are whole-grain cereals, egg yolks, seeds, and green vegetables.

**Medical Durable Power of Attorney**: A document that designates an agent or proxy to make healthcare decisions for a patient who is unable to do so.

**Melanoma**: The most serious of the types of skin cancer.

**Metastatic**: The spread of tumor cells to distant body parts.

**Morphine (Morphine Sulfate)**: A habit-forming narcotic drug that reduces pain without the loss of consciousness.

**Narcotic**: A habit-forming drug that induces euphoria, mood changes, and alters perception to pain.

**Nasogastric (NG) tube**: A narrow plastic tube that is passed through the nose, esophagus, then into the stomach.

**Natural killer (NK) cells**: Important white blood cells that are evaluated in immunotherapy to determine the toxic effects on cells.

**Nurse anesthetist**: A registered nurse with advanced education and training in nurse anesthesia who administers anesthesia and manages the care of the patient in surgical situations.

**Nutritionist**: A specialist who deals in the science of promoting health and nourishment of human beings through a balanced diet.

**Oncologist**: A physician who specializes in the diagnosis and treatment of abnormal tumors (benign or malignant), but is particularly involved with cancer treatments.

**Ophthalmologist**: A physician who specializes in the care of the eyes.

**Over-the-counter (OTC) drug**: A drug available without a prescription which generally is considered safe for consumers if properly used.

**Palpitations**: An awareness of the heartbeat when the heart is beating harder and/or faster.

**Patient Controlled Analgesia (PCA)**: A device that allows patients to administer their own pain medication in a safe and accurate dosage as prescribed by the physician.

**Patient Self-Determination Act**: A 1991 Federal act that requires hospitals, nursing homes, home health agencies, hospices, and health maintenance organizations that receive Medicaid or Medicare funds to inform patients of their rights to accept or refuse medical treatment and to prepare advance directives for health care.

**Physiological**: Characteristic of body functions and vital processes.

**Potassium**: A mineral that maintains heartbeat, water balance, and nerve function. Sources are bananas, milk, salmon, and potatoes.

**Preferred Provider Organization (PPO)**: A comprehensive healthcare plan offered to employees that allows them to choose their own physicians and hospitals within certain limits.

**Prothrombin time**: A test that measures the activity of clotting factors in the blood prior to surgery.

**Psychiatrist**: A physician who specializes in the treatment of mental, emotional, or behavioral problems.

**Psychologist**: A specialist in the science dealing with the mind and with the mental and emotional processes.

**Rheumatoid arthritis**: A chronic disease characterized by inflammation, pain, and swelling of the joints that can lead to deformities.

**Sedation**: The use of a drug to calm a person.

**Sodium**: A mineral that maintains water balance in the body and is involved in nerve and muscle function. Excessive amounts can cause fluid retention and increased blood pressure in some individuals. It is found in canned soups, meat tenderizer, garlic/onion salts, frozen dinners, sauerkraut, dill pickles, ham, frankfurters, and tomato juice.

**Steroids**: Any of a large number of hormonal substances with a similar basic chemical structure, that are often produced in the adrenal gland or by the ovary or testis and are used to treat some diseases.

**Stress test**: A test that measures the function of a system of the body when subjected to carefully controlled amounts of physiological stress. It is often used to check heart or respiratory function.

**Surgeon**: A physician who performs operations.

**Syphilis**: A sexually transmitted, infectious disease caused by a bacterium, that if left untreated, can lead to the degeneration of heart, bone, and nerve tissue.

**Systemic**: Affecting the entire organism or bodily system.

**T-cells**: A type of lymphocyte (white blood cell) that plays an important role in the body's immune system.

**Tannins (tannic acid)**: Chemicals that occur in plants, in the barks of trees, and in tea.

**Therapist**: A specialist who is involved in the treatment of any disease or abnormal physical or mental condition.

**Toxic**: Pertaining to or having the effect of a poison.

**Ulcer**: A crater-like lesion of the skin or mucous membrane resulting from some inflammatory, infectious, or malignant process.

**Ultrasound**: A diagnostic technique in which high frequency sound waves (inaudible to the human ear) are passed into the body; the reflected echoes are detected and analyzed to build a picture of the internal organs or of a fetus in the uterus.

**Urinalysis**: A battery of tests on a patient's urine, including measurements of the urine's physical characteristics, microscopic examination, and chemical testing to check kidney function or urinary problems.

**Virus**: The smallest known type of infectious agent that causes infections, ranging from colds to serious diseases like AIDS and probably some types of cancers.

**Visualization**: The experience of forming mental images of something that is not present to the sight.

**Vital signs**: The measurements of pulse rate, respiration rate, body temperature, and blood pressure that are clues to diseases and evaluate a patient's progress.

**Vitamins**: Any of a group of organic substances essential in small quantities to normal metabolism that are found naturally in food and sometimes produced synthetically.

**Vitamin A**: A fat-soluble vitamin that assists the formation and maintenance of skin, mucous membranes, bones, and teeth and is important to the visual process of the eye. Sources are carrots, dark green leafy vegetables, sweet potato, cantaloupe, winter squash, liver, and milk.

**Vitamin B-complex**: Water-soluble vitamins of which some are $B_1$ (thiamine), $B_2$ (riboflavin), $B_3$ (niacin), $B_6$ (pyridoxine), $B_{12}$, biotin, and folic acid. They are active in providing the body with energy by converting carbohydrates into glucose, which the body "burns" to produce energy, and they are necessary for the functioning of the nervous system. Sources are whole-grain/fortified cereals, brewer's yeast, sunflower seeds, liver, wheat germ, and milk.

**Vitamin C**: A water-soluble vitamin that assists in maintaining the supportive material in tissue, helps in wound healing, and promotes iron absorption. Sources are citrus fruits, broccoli, cantaloupe, potato, green pepper, tomato, peas, and spinach.

**Vitamin E**: A fat-soluble vitamin that allows Vitamin A and unsaturated fatty acids to perform their specific functions and prevents cell damage due to excess oxygen. Sources are whole grains, seeds, margarine, polyunsaturated vegetable oils, and peanuts.

**X-ray**: Form of invisible electromagnetic energy that is used to produce images of bones, organs, and internal tissues.

**Zinc**: An essential trace mineral needed to make several enzymes and insulin, that is important in healing wounds and burns, and is related to the normal absorption and action of vitamins. Sources are whole-grain/fortified cereals, veal, turkey, liver, shrimp, lamb, and lentils.

## REFERENCES

Anderson, Judith V., and Marian R. Van Nierop, eds. *Basic Nutrition Facts: A Nutrition Reference*. East Lansing, MI: Co-operative Extension Service, Michigan State University, 1989.

Anderson, Kenneth N., Lois E. Anderson, and Walter D. Glanze, eds. *Mosby's Medical Dictionary*. Chicago, IL: Mosby, 1994.

Clayman, Charles B., ed. *The American Medical Association Encyclopedia of Medicine.* New York, NY: Random House, 1989.

McEvoy, Gerald, K., Kathy Litvak, and Olin H. Welsh, Jr., eds. *American Hospital Formulatory Service 96 Drug Information.* Bethesda, MD: The American Society of Health-System Pharmacists, Inc., 1996.

Pyle, Vera. *Current Medical Terminology.* Modesto, CA: Health Professions Institute, 1996.

Westley, Gregory J., Edna V. Berger, and Jeffrey Schaefer, eds. *Physicians' Desk Reference (PDR).* Montvale, NJ: Medical Economics Company, 1996.

Wilson, Loren Stevenson, and Brian Dennison, eds. *Mosby's Diagnostic and Laboratory Test Reference.* Chicago, IL: Mosby, 1995.

# SELF-HELP GROUPS

*T*he goal of a self-help group is to empower its members with the tools necessary to make adjustments needed to continue a life of dignity and independence.

Self-help groups share a common health concern, provide non-judgmental emotional support for each other, and share specialized information. They use peer leaders, may reach out to professionals for resources, and increase public awareness and knowledge by sharing their unique and relevant information.

The following health groups would be helpful to people having surgery. This list is printed with the permission of the American Self-Help Clearinghouse, Northwest Covenant Medical Center, 25 Pocono Road, Denville, NJ 07834-2995, (201) 625-7101.

**American Liver Foundation**: National. 24 chapters. Founded 1976. Dedicated to fighting all liver diseases through research, education, and patient self-help groups. Chapters organized and operated by lay volunteers. Quarterly newsletter, chapter development guidelines. Write: 1425 Pompton Ave., Cedar Grove, NJ 07009. Call: (201) 256-2550 or (800) 223-0179.

**Center for Attitudinal Healing, The**: National. 100+ affiliates. Founded 1975. Support programs for children, adolescents and adults facing their own, or a family member's life-threatening illness, loss, and grief. All services free of charge. Quarterly newsletter. Write: 33 Buchanan, Sausalito, CA 94965. Call: (415) 331-6161. Fax: (415) 331-4545. E-mail: home123@aol.com

**International Association of Laryngectomees**: Int'l. 285 chapters. Founded 1952. Acts as a bridge starting before laryngectomy surgery through rehabilitation, and for practical and emotional support. Newsletter. Chapter development guidelines. Write: Int'l Assn. of Laryngectomees, 7440 N. Shadeland Ave., #100, Indianapolis, IN 46250. Call: (317) 570-4568. Fax: (317) 570-4570.

**Let's Face It**: National. U.S. branch of Int'l. Founded 1987. Network for people with facial disfigurement. Phone help, pen, and phone pals. Referrals to resources. Annual 50-page resource list with over 190 resources available by sending 9x12 $3 stamped self-addressed envelope with interest (child or adult). Write: Let's Face It, P.O. Box 29972, Bellingham, WA 98228-1972. Call: Betsy Wilson at (360) 676-7325. E-mail: letsfaceit@faceit.org. Website: http://www.faceit.org/~letsfaceit/

**Make Today Count**: National. Founded 1974. Mutual support and discussion for persons facing a life-threatening illness. Open to relatives and friends. Chapter development guidelines. Write: c/o St. John's Regional Health Center, Mid-America Cancer Center, 1235 E. Cherokee, Springfield, MO 65804-2263. Call: Connie Zimmerman at (800) 432-2273 (Mid-America Cancer Services). Fax: (417) 888-7426.

**Man To Man Program**: National. 250 affiliated groups. Founded 1990. Support and education for men with prostate cancer to enable them to better understand their options and to make informed decisions. Phone support, information, and referrals, support group meetings, newsletter. Help in starting new groups. Contact: the American Cancer Society at (800) ACS-2345; Website: http://www.cancer.org

**National Chronic Pain Outreach Association, Inc.**: National network. Founded 1980. Clearinghouse for information about chronic pain and pain management. Aims at increasing public awareness and decreasing the stigma of chronic pain. Provides kit to develop local support groups, professional education, quarterly magazine, and other materials. Dues $25.00/yr. Write: 7979 Old Georgetown Rd. #100, Bethesda, MD 20814. Call: (301) 652-4948. Fax: (301) 907-0745.

**National Coalition for Cancer Survivorship**: National. 400 member organizations. Founded 1986. Clearinghouse for information on survivorship, including support groups nationwide, insurance, and employment issues. Advocacy for cancer survivors. Assistance in starting cancer support and networking systems. Newsletter. Conferences. Write: 1010 Wayne Ave., 5th Fl., Suite #505, Silver Spring, MD 20910. Call (301) 650-8868.

**National Empowerment Center**: Mental health consumer-run center that provides information on local self-help resources and upcoming conferences. Also provides networking, conference calls and workshops. Write: 20 Ballard Rd., Lawrence, MA 01843. Call: (508) 685-1518 or (800) POWER-2-U. Fax: (508) 681-6426.

**National Mental Health Consumers Self-Help Clearinghouse**: Consumer self-help resource information geared towards meeting the individual and group needs of mental health consumers. Assistance in advocacy, listings of publications, on-site consultations, training, educational events. Funded by Center of Mental Health Services. Write: Nat'l MH Consumers Self-Help Clearinghouse, 1211 Chestnut St., #1000, Philadelphia, PA 19107-4103. Call: (800) 553-4-KEY. Fax: (215) 636-6310. Website: http://www.libertynet.org/~mha/cl_house.html

**United Ostomy Association**: National. 580 chapters. Founded 1962. Dedicated to helping every person with an ostomy and related surgeries return to normal living. Provides education, support to local chapters, and national identity. Chapter development help, visitation program, magazine. Write: 36 Executive Park #120, Irvine, CA 92614. Call: (800) 826-0826 or (714) 660-8624.

**Us Too**: International. 400 affiliated groups. Founded 1990. Mutual support, information, and education for prostate cancer patients, their families, and friends. Provides newsletter, information and referrals, phone support, assistance in starting new groups. Write: 930 N. York Rd., Suite 50, Hinsdale, IL 60521-2993. Call: (800) 808-7866 or (630) 323-1002.

**Well Spouse Foundation**: International. 90 support groups. Founded 1988. Provides support and information to the well spouses of the chronically ill, educators, human service professionals and the public about the needs of spousal caregivers. Bi-monthly newsletter. Round Robins. Guidelines and assistance available for starting new groups. Write: Well Spouse Fdn., 610 Lexington Ave., #814, New York, NY 10022-6005. Call: (800) 838-0879 or (212) 644-1241. Fax: (212) 644-1338. E-mail: wellspouse@aol.com

**Y-ME National Breast Cancer Organization**: National. 19 affiliated groups. Founded 1978. Information and peer support for breast cancer patients and their families during all stages of the disease. Community outreach to educate people on early detection. Hotline, newsletter, group development guidelines, conferences. Write: 212 W. Van Buren St., 4th Fl., Chicago, IL 60607-3908. Call: (800) 221-2141 (day) or (312) 986-8228 (24 hrs).

# NATIONAL RESOURCES
## (INCLUDING WEBSITES)

**American Association of Retired Persons (AARP):**
(800) 424-3410    http://www.aarp.org/

**American Board of Medical Specialties:**
(800) 776-2378    http://www.webcom.com/abms/

**American Cancer Society:**
(800) 227-2345    http://www.cancer.org/

**American College of Surgeons:**
(312) 664-4050    http://www.facs.org/

**American Heart Association:**
(800) 242-8721    http://www.americanheart.org/

**American Hospital Association:**
(312) 422-3000
http://www.social.com/health/nhic/data/hr0600/hr0654.html

**American Institute for Cancer Research:**
(800) 843-8114, (202) 328-7744 in D.C.
http://www.aicr.org/

**American Institute for Preventive Medicine:**
(810) 539-1800
http://wellness.uwsp.edu/nfla/members/Powell.htm

**American Lung Association:**
(212) 315-8700    http://www.lungusa.org/

**American Medical Association:**
(312) 464-5000
http://www.ama-assn.org/home/amahome.htm

**American Red Cross**:
(703) 206-7502    http://www.crossnet.org/

**American Self-Help Clearinghouse**:
(201) 625-7101    http://www.cmhc.com/selfhelp/

**Center for Patient Advocacy**:
(800) 846-7444    http://www.patientadvocacy.org/

**Choice in Dying**:
(212 ) 366-5540    http://www.choices.org/

**Exceptional Cancer Patients (ECaP)**:
(860) 343-5950
http://www.hmt.com/cyp/nonprof/ecap/index.html

**Food and Drug Administration**:
(301) 443-1544    http://www.fda.gov/

**Food and Nutrition Information Center**:
(301) 504-5719    http://www.nalusda.gov/fnic/

**Med Help International**:
(407) 253-9048    http://www.medhelp.org/home.htm

**Medicare Telephone Hotline**:
(800) 638-6833

**National Alliance of Breast Cancer Organizations**:
(800) 719-9154    http://nysernet.org/bcic/numbers/nabco.html

**National Association for Home Care**:
(202) 547-7424    http://www.nahc.org/home.html

**National Cancer Institute**:
(800) 422-6237    http://www.nci.nih.gov/mab/hnc.htm

**National Coalition for Cancer Survivorship**:
(301) 650-8868
http://www.access.digex.net/~mkragen/cansearch.html

**National Consumers League**:
(202) 835-3323    http://www.aoa.dhhs.gov/aoa/dir/148.html

**National Health Information Center**:
(800) 336-4797, (301) 565-4167 in Maryland
http://nhic-nt.health.org/

**National Hospice Foundation**:
(703) 516-4928    http://www.nho.org/foundati.htm

**National Institutes of Health**:
(301) 496-4000    http://www.nih.gov/

**National Insurance Consumer Helpline**:
(800) 942-4242

**National Wellness Institute**:
(800) 243-8694    http://www.wellnessnwi.org/nwa.htm

**Office of Disease Prevention and Health Promotion**:
(202) 205-8611    http://odphp.oash.dhhs.gov/

**People's Medical Society**:
(610) 770-1670
http://www.social.com/health/nhic/data/hr2000/hr2079.html

**Visiting Nurse Associations of America**:
(303) 753-0218    http://www.aoa.dhhs.gov/aoa/dir/226.html

## REFERENCES

Ankrapp, Betty, and Sara Nell Di Lima, eds. *1996 National Health Directory.* Gaithersburg, Maryland: An Aspen Publication, 1996.

Cancer Research Institute. *Cancer Research Institute HelpBook.* New York: Cancer Research Institute, 1991.

Mackenzie, Leslie and Amy Lignor, eds. *1994-The Complete Directory for People With Chronic Illness.* Lakeville, CT: Grey House Publishing, 1994.

Mackenzie, Leslie, and Amy Lignor. *1995/96-The Complete Directory for People With Disabilities.* Lakeville, CT: Grey House Publishing, 1995.

# BIBLIOGRAPHY

## DOCTOR / CANCER / HOSPITAL / SURGERY

Altenberg, Henry E. *Holistic Medicine*. New York, NY: Japan Publications, Inc., 1992.

Altman, Roberta. *The Prostate Answer*. New York, NY: A Time Warner Company, 1993.

Baker, Robert W. *Successful Surgery: A Doctor's Mind-Body Guide to Help You Through Surgery*. New York, NY: Pocket Books, 1996.

Bradley III, Edward L. *A Patient's Guide to Surgery*. Yonkers, NY: Consumer Reports Books, 1994.

Cafferty, Michael E. *Managed Care and You: The Consumer Guide to Managing Your Health Care*. New York, NY: McGraw Hill, Inc., 1995.

*How to Find the Best Doctors, Hospitals, and HMO'S for You and Your Family: Pocket Guide*. New York, NY: Castle Connolly Medical Ltd., 1995.

Chopra, Deepak. *Quantum Healing: Exploring the Frontiers of Mind/Body Medicine*. New York, NY: Bantam Books, 1989.

Evans, Richard A. *Making the Right Choice: Treatment Options in Cancer Surgery*. Garden City Park, NY: Avery Publishing Group, Inc. 1995.

Gelbard, Martin. *Solving Prostate Problems*. New York, NY: A Fireside Book, 1995.

Goleman, Daniel, and Joel Gurin, eds. *Mind, Body Medicine: How to Use Your Mind For Better Health.* Yonkers, NY: Consumer Reports Books, 1993.

Greenberg, Martin D. *Hysterectomy: Making a Choice.* New York, NY: The Body Press/Perigee, 1993.

Griffith, Winter H. *The Complete Guide to Symptoms, Illness, & Surgery.* New York, NY: The Body Press/Perigee, 1995.

Haas, Adelaide and Susan L. Puretz. *The Women's Guide to Hysterectomy.* Berkeley, CA: Celestial Arts, 1995.

Hardt, Barbara, and Katharine Halkin. *The New Way to Take Charge of Your Medical Treatment: A Patient's Guide.* New York, NY: Madison Books, 1995.

Huddleston, Peggy. *Prepare for Surgery, Heal Faster: A Guide of Mind-Body Techniques.* North Cambridge, MA: Angel River Press, 1996.

Inlander, Charles B., and Ed Weiner. *Take This Book to the Hospital With You: A Consumer Guide to Surviving Your Hospital Stay.* Allentown, PA: The People's Medical Society, 1985, 1991, 1995.

Keating, Karen. *Take Charge of Your Hospital Stay: A "Start Smart" Guide for Patients and Care Partners.* New York, NY: Insight Books, 1994.

Komarnicky, Lydia, and Anne Rosenberg. *What to Do if You Get Breast Cancer.* New York, NY: Little Brown and Company, 1995.

Korda, Michael. *Man-to-Man: Surviving Prostate Cancer.* New York, NY: Random House, 1996.

Margolis, Simeon. *Johns Hopkins Symptoms and Remedies.* New York, NY: Rebus, 1995.

Marks, Sheldon. *Prostate & Cancer: A Family Guide to Diagnosis, Treatment & Survival.* Tucson, AZ: Fisher Books, 1995.

McCall, Timothy B. *Examining Your Doctor.* New York, NY: A Birch Lane Book, 1995.

McDougal, W. Scott. *Prostate Disease.* New York, NY: Times Book, 1996.

Miller, Jr., Ryle, and Geoffrey G. McCullen. *Hip and Knee Replacement: A Patient's Guide.* New York, NY: W.W. Norton & Company, 1996.

Olivotto, Ivo. *Intelligent Patient Guide to Breast Cancer: All You Need to Know to Take an Active Part in Your Treatment.* Vancouver, British Columbia, Canada: Intelligent Patient Guide, 1995.

Schwartz, Marti Ann. *Listen to Me, Doctor: Taking Charge of Your Own Health Care.* Aspen, CO: MacMurray & Beck, Inc., 1995.

Shapiro, Kenneth A. *Dying & Living: One Man's Life With Cancer.* Austin, TX: University of Texas Press, 1985.

Shaw, Michael, ed. *Everything You Needed to Know About Medical Tests.* Springhouse, PA: Springhouse Corporation, 1996.

Shulman, Julius. *Cataracts: From Diagnosis to Recovery-The Complete Guide for Patients and Families.* New York, NY: St. Martin's Press, 1993.

Swirsky, Joan, and Barbara Balaban. *The Breast Cancer Handbook.* New York, NY: Harper Perennial, 1994.

Tyberg, Theodore, and Kenneth Rothaus. *The Insider's Survival Guide to Your Hospital, Your Doctor, The Nursing Staff and Your Bill!* New York, NY: Hearst Books, 1995.

Virog, Irene. *We're All in This Together.* Kansas City, MO: Andrews and McMeel, 1995.

Walsh, Patrick, and Janet Farrar Worthington. *The Prostate: A Guide for Men and the Women Who Love Them.* Baltimore, MD: The Johns Hopkins University Press, 1995.

Youngson, Robert, and the Diagram Group. *The Surgery Book.* New York, NY: St. Martin's Press, 1993.

## HEALTH / NUTRITION / HEALING

Anderson, Greg. *Healing Wisdom: Wit, Insight & Inspiration for Anyone Facing Illness.* New York, NY: A Dutton Book, 1994.

Appleton, Nancy. *Lick the Sugar Habit.* New York, NY: Avery Publishing Group, Inc., 1988.

Balch, James F., and Phyllis A. Balch. *Prescription for Nutritional Healing.* New York, NY: Avery Publishing Group, Inc., 1990.

Benson, Herbert, and Mary Stark. *Timeless Healing: The Power and Biology of Belief.* New York, NY: A Fireside Book, 1996.

Carlson, Karen J. *The Harvard Guide to Women's Health.* Cambridge, MA: Harvard University Press, 1996.

Chopra, Deepak. *Journey Into Healing: Awakening the Wisdom Within You.* New York, NY: Harmony Books, 1994.

Davidson, James, and Jan Ninebrenner. *In Touch With Your Breasts.* Waco, TX: WRS Publishing, 1995.

Doukas, David J., and William Reichel. *Planning for Uncertainty: A Guide to Living Wills and Other Advance Directives for Health Care.* Baltimore, MD: The Johns Hopkins University Press, 1993.

Epstein, Gerald. *Healing Visualization: Creating Health Through Imagery.* New York, NY: Bantam Books, 1989.

Feinstein, Alice, ed. *Women's Health Advisor.* Emmaus, PA: Rodale Press, 1995.

Gershoff, Stanley. *The Tufts University Guide to Total Nutrition.* New York, NY: Harper Perennial, 1996.

Healy, Bernadine. *A New Prescription for Women's Health.* New York, NY: Viking, 1995.

Kessler, David. *The Doctor's Complete Guide to Healing Foods.* New York, NY: Berkley Books, 1996.

Klein, Allen. *The Healing Power of Humor.* New York, NY: G.P. Putnam's Sons, 1989.

Love, Susan M. *Dr. Susan Love's Breast Book.* New York, NY: Addison-Wesley Publishing Company, 1990, 1991, 1995.

Powell, Don R. *Self-Care: Your Family Guide to Symptoms and How to Treat Them.* Allentown, PA: People's Medical Society, 1996.

Roberts, H.J. *Aspartame (Nutrasweet) Is It Safe?* Philadelphia, PA: The Charles Press, 1990.

Rybacki, James J., and James W. Long. *The Essential Guide to Prescription Drugs.* New York, NY: Harper Perennial, 1996.

Siegel, Bernie S. *How to Live Between Office Visits: A Guide to Life, Love and Health.* New York, NY: HarperCollins Publishers, 1993.

Siegel, Bernie S. *Love, Medicine & Miracles.* New York, NY: Harper Perennial, 1986, 1990.

Siegel, Bernie S. *Peace, Love & Healing: Bodymind Communication and the Path to Self Healing.* New York, NY: Harper Perennial, 1989, 1990.

Spratt, John S., Rhonda L. Hawley, and Robert E. Hoyle, eds. *Home Health Care: Principles and Practices.* Delray Beach, FL: GR/St. Lucie Press, 1997.

Terry, Paul E., David Abelson, and Allan Kind. *Take Charge of Your Health: A Practical Guide to Everyday Decisions.* St. Louis, MO: Park Nicollet Medical Foundation, 1995.

University of California at Berkeley Wellness Letter, eds. *The New Wellness Encyclopedia.* New York, NY: Houghton Mifflin Company, 1995.

Weil, Andrew. *Health and Healing.* New York, NY: Houghton Mifflin Company, 1983, 1988, 1995.

Weil, Andrew. *Spontaneous Healing.* New York, NY: Alfred A. Knopf, Inc., 1995.

Wertheimer, Neil., ed. *Total Health for Men: How to Prevent and Treat Health Problems That Trouble Men the Most.* Emmaus, PA: Rodale Press, 1995.

White, Barbara J., and Edward J. Madara. *The Self-Help Sourcebook: Finding and Forming Mutual Aid Self-Help Groups.* Denville, NJ: Northwest Covenant Medical Center, 1986, 1988, 1990, 1992, 1995.

## STRESS / COPING / FAMILY / GRIEVING

Eliot, Robert S. *From Stress to Strength: How to Lighten Your Load and Save Your Life.* New York, NY: Bantam Books, 1994.

Farhi, Donna. *The Breathing Book.* New York, NY: Henry Holt and Company, 1996.

Hart, Archibald, D. *Stress and Your Child.* Dallas, TX: Word Publishing, 1992.

Helmstetter, Shad. *What to Say When You Talk to Yourself.* New York, NY: Pocket Books, 1986.

Kent, Howard. *Breathe Better.* Allentown, PA: A People's Medical Society Book, 1997.

Lark, Susan M. *Anxiety & Stress Self-Help Book.* Berkeley, CA: Celestial Arts, 1993, 1996

Olson, B. Kaye. *Energy Secrets For Tired Mothers on the Run.* Deerfield Beach, FL: Health Communications, Inc., 1993.

Powell, Trevor. *Free Yourself From Harmful Stress.* New York, NY: DK Publishing, Inc., 1997.

Siegler, Ava L. *What Should I Tell the Kids?: A Parent's Guide to Real Problems in the Real World.* New York, NY: A Plume Book, 1993.

Stearns, Ann Kaiser. *Coming Back: Rebuilding Lives After Crisis and Loss.* New York, NY: Ballantine Books, 1988.

Williams, Redford, and Virginia Williams. *Anger Kills: Seventeen Strategies for Controlling the Hostility That Can Harm Your Health.* New York, NY: Harper Perennial, 1993.

# INDEX

# ORDER INFORMATION

## *Give the gift of health to someone you care about!*

Order **Surgery and Recovery** from your bookstore.

If unavailable at your bookstore, please send $12.95 plus $3.50 for shipping and handling for each book. If five or more copies, $2.00 s/h per book. Michigan residents add 6% sales tax.
Send_____ books.

Also available from author, Kaye Olson:
Audio book-tape: **Energy Secrets for Women on the Run.** Two cassettes, approximately two hours, $14.95, plus $3.50 for shipping and handling for each audio book-tape. If five or more copies, $2.00 s/h per tape. Michigan residents add 6% sales tax.
Send_____tapes.

PLEASE PRINT

Name: _____

Address: _____  Apt # _____

City: _____  State: ____  Zip: _____

Send check or money order (payable to Working Well) plus above information to:

> **Working Well**
> **P.O. Box 335**
> **DeWitt, MI  48820**